THE FIBROMYALGIA CHALLENGE

ALICE MOWERY BURNWORTH, CKBD

ISBN:1517346770
ISBN-13:9781517346775

PREFACE

My one goal in writing this book is to help my readers lead more productive and symptom-free lives. Its purpose is to help them meet the challenges that we who have autoimmune problems must face daily.

I have based my book on over ten years of research and on my own experiences of living with fibromyalgia and other autoimmune disorders, some of which began as early as my late teens.

My journey has not been without complications as I have had to rewrite the book three times in all. I lost it once to the mysteries of "cyberspace"…Even the expert that looked for it buried somewhere within my computer could only find three pages of the book.

The next time I lost it to "cyber pirates" who destroyed my book and years of family pictures when I would not come up with ransom.

I am very pleased to offer my book to you now! It is my hope that it will encourage you to set up a healing program that you find easy to live with; one that fits you personally.

CONTENTS

ACKNOWLEDGMENTS

I wish to thank my family and friends who have encouraged me to not give up. In the process of writing this book, I have lost it once to the mysteries of cyberspace, and once to cybernet piracy. It has been a labor of love and dedication to those out there looking for encouragement and help from one who has tread the same path they now are on to the recovery of a happy life in spite of a dysfunctional autoimmune system. May God bless your journey. ~Alice Mowery Burnworth~

CHAPTER 1
WHAT IS FIBROMYALGIA?

"You Cannot See Pain, Mental Fog and Fatigue"

"What is fibromyalgia?" This is an important question that many fibromyalgia sufferers find difficult to answer. They may be able to describe how it makes them feel, but find it difficult to answer this simple question when it is put to them by someone who has never heard of fibromyalgia. Please bear with me as we will begin by discussing a little of what fibromyalgia is and a little of what fibromyalgia is not.

People may not be able to tell, by looking at you, that you spent your entire night in pain, unable to sleep; or that when you did sleep, you were subconsciously aware of the pain. I suppose, in some ways we are fortunate to not look as badly as we sometimes feel.

According to the Cleveland clinic, "Fibromyalgia is a syndrome rather than a disease. A syndrome is a collection of signs, symptoms, and medical problems that tend to occur together but are not related to a specific, identifiable cause. A disease, on the other hand, has specific causes with recognizable signs and symptoms."

A report put out by the University of Maryland Medical Center stated: "Fibromyalgia can be difficult to diagnose. It can take 5 years for the average person with the condition to finally get a diagnosis, and as many as three out of every four people with fibromyalgia remain undiagnosed."

Though it is not a life-threatening illness by itself; persons who have fibromyalgia almost always have autoimmune disease symptoms overlapping or coexisting with fibromyalgia. Whatever the reason may truly be, people who suffer from fibromyalgia appear to have challenged immune systems.

A challenged immune system makes you susceptible to infections, contagions and other health risks that the average person might easily fight off. For this reason, you should support your immune system at all times with proper diet and a prescribed exercise program.

DIAGNOSIS

There are 18 possible "tender points" on the human body commonly used for diagnosis of fibromyalgia. The severe pain caused by simply applying pressure to these points can even be a surprise to the person being examined, who possibly did not know such pain could be experienced by simply applying pressure to these parts of their bodies.

These tender points are used in the diagnosis of fibromyalgia because they are located in the same identical sites on the bodies of everyone who has fibromyalgia. Generally, doctors require at least 11 of the 18 sites to be very painful when firmly pressed for the diagnosis of fibromyalgia.

But it is essential that doctors base their diagnosis on health history as well as tender points. In this way, they may be able to reduce the fibromyalgia symptoms their patients are experiencing by treating these other existing health problems as well.

WIDESPREAD PAIN

Fibromyalgia is a life-changing condition that affects the fibrous tissues, ligaments, muscles and tendons; this causes widespread pain, fatigue and stiffness throughout the body; though the most commonly reported areas of pain are usually found to be in the neck, shoulders and hips.

Though there have been many speculative theories as to the cause of this widespread pain, recent studies reveal that because of the lack of proper blood supply and the nutrients that it carries to the muscles, the lactic acid and waste products do not get washed away and the tears in the muscles do not get properly repaired.

This causes scar tissue to form on the muscles. The resulting scar tissue on the muscles and the buildup of lactic acid in the muscles are greatly responsible for the pain you experience.
Read more in the chapter, "The Collagen Connection".

Fibromyalgia pain symptoms may vary from one time to another; affecting various areas of the body throughout the day. Often the pain will seem to stay isolated in certain areas for days at a time and then at other times it will affect one part of your body for now, a completely different part an hour later and so on and on throughout the day. This quite often causes changes in your daily routine, and plans that have to be cancelled at the last minute (very frustrating for you and for anyone counting on you).

Besides actual muscle pain, There are various other ways that fibromyalgia can affect the muscles and tissues of the body such as:

- A tendency to have tendonitis and bursitis pain involved along with fibromyalgia pain.

- It is common for some people to experience symptoms akin to neuropathy in the feet, legs, arms or face. This "neuropathy" may be described as numbness, tingling (vibrating), or burning feeling. This is a very unsettling sensation...as sometimes you can actually feel you are standing or sitting on a vibrator. However, if you are tested for neuropathy, do not be surprised if the test results are negative. Fibromyalgia mimics many illnesses.

- There can be a very deep sense of exhaustion comparable to the fatigue described in Chronic Fatigue Syndrome (CFS).

Is Fibromyalgia a Progressive Illness?

Although fibromyalgia is not supposed to be a progressive illness, there are several kinds of fibromyalgia pain and the intensity of fibromyalgia pain is often affected by outside influences and associated illnesses. If you develop health problems (especially ones typically known to increase fibromyalgia symptoms) then you will be more apt to experience more flare-ups, pain etc. than you were before. A good example of this is menopause…some women may see an increase in the intensity of their symptoms just before and during menopause (and often continuing afterwards).

The more intense pain is usually felt only during flare-ups, but there are some people who seem to be more prone to flare ups than others are, causing these more intense pains to seem almost a constant thing in their lives.

There are people diagnosed with fibromyalgia that may only experience bouts of stiffness, muscle ache and fatigue. Then suddenly, their symptoms may become extremely magnified to the point of being disabling. This could cause you to suspect fibromyalgia of being a progressive syndrome. But fibromyalgia is not a stand-alone problem. Anything that affects your health and well-being will affect your fibromyalgia symptoms…even weather and seasonal changes.

In 2002, a study was conducted in Cordoba, Argentina, where there are four distinct seasons every year. The study involved fibromyalgia sufferers and a healthy control group and aimed to find out whether pain symptoms could be linked to specific weather changes.

Participants were asked to rate their pain symptoms on a scale from one to ten, every day for 12 months. After 12 months, these symptoms were correlated to weather patterns for the entire year. Researchers found that pain symptoms of the participants with fibromyalgia correlated directly to weather changes. Specifically, pain increased as temperatures fell and atmospheric pressure increased.

The healthy control group did not show any correlation between pain and weather patterns.

So though fibromyalgia pain is not necessarily predictable; it definitely is influenced by our general state of health as well as outside influences.

MEMORY PROBLEMS

Fibromyalgia patients often have cognitive problems commonly referred to as "fibro fog". Fibro fog is the terminology used for "fuzzy thinking and mental confusion". It seems to be worse when there is more pain and exhaustion involved.

The time of day can also be a deciding factor in the degree of fibro fog experienced. Some people experience fibro fog at its worst when they first awaken, while some people seem to experience it more at the end of a long tiring day.

The depth of pain, exhaustion, and fibro fog can be affected by such things as:
- stress (good or bad stress)
- poor sleep habits
- over-exertion
- allergy
- dietary changes
- weather changes

Fibromyalgia can cause memory problems so troublesome that some people have even been misdiagnosed as having Alzheimer's disease while going through some of the more difficult phases of FMS. It is so disturbing to find yourself drawing a complete blank about common everyday things that you would be expected to know. You find yourself secretly hoping that one of these temporary memory lapses will not embarrass you in public.

Fortunately, just as flare-ups come and go, so the worst of the memory problems usually come and go also.

ASSOCIATED SLEEP DISORDERS

There are various forms of sleep problems common to fibromyalgia such as:
- "non-restorative sleep" (feeling worse upon awakening than before going to sleep),
- sleep apnea,
- daytime sleepiness
- "Sleep attacks" similar to narcolepsy (but not causing paresthesia of the muscles) have been known to affect some

people. This is when the eyes are active but the body is not active (such as when driving or reading). This can affect anyone to a degree, but with fibromyalgia it can cause sleep deprivation symptoms comparable to those of narcolepsy. These are often preceded by imagining a loud noise in the head or by a sort of "dream-like hallucination" before leading into the sudden sleep attack.

EXTENDED SYMPTOMS

Although persons with fibromyalgia may often experience the following list of symptoms, you should not take them for granted. Fibromyalgia can mimic many serious illnesses, so it is important that you bring any *new symptoms*, such as those listed below, to your physician's attention.

- Depression…Chronic pain can affect an individual's life by causing an imbalance in the serotonin levels…just as imbalanced serotonin levels can be linked to occasional bouts of depression.
- Mood swings
- Falling asleep during daytime activities
- Headaches
- Muscle weakness
- Anxiety attacks
- Adrenal exhaustion
- Short term memory problems
- Fuzzy headedness
- Forgetfulness
- Heel pain
- Bruised feeling
- Often using wrong words
- Hands feel swelled (but they aren't)
- Persistent rashes
- Severe itching (sometimes over whole body)
- Sensitivity to light
- Mild butterfly rash on the face (of the lupus type…but not Lupus)
- Sensitivity to smells

- Sensitivity to temperature
- Dry eyes
- Dry mouth
- Dizziness
- Ringing in the ears
- Hair loss
- Repeated yeast infections
- Knee and leg pain
- Sensitivity to noise
- Sudden unexplainable irritability
- Foot pain (can even feel like you have broken bones in your foot)
- Sleep attacks especially if sitting down (for example: when reading or driving, and occasionally when playing piano or working at the computer)

RELATED ILLNESSES AND DISORDERS

Fibromyalgia can seemingly develop on its own, in conjunction with other autoimmune illnesses, or with various other disorders (such as the ones listed below). By simply reducing these symptoms, you can often reduce your overall fibromyalgia symptoms also. Likewise, an increase in the following disorders can increase your overall fibromyalgia symptoms considerably:

- Adrenal fatigue
- Arthritis
- Bursitis
- Carpal tunnel syndrome
- Celiac disease
- Chemical sensitivity
- Epstein Barr Syndrome
- Estrogen Dominance
- GERD
- Heartburn
- Hypoglycemia
- Irritable bladder syndrome
- IBS (irritable bowel syndrome)
- Lyme disease
- Lupus

- Myofascial pain (very similar to fibromyalgia)
- Narcolepsy symptoms (often improves with age)
- Paresthesia of the muscles (painful gout, tingling and numbness)
- Peripheral neuropathy
- Premature menopause
- Menopause
- Raynaud's phenomena
- Rheumatoid arthritis
- Restless leg syndrome
- Sleep apnea
- Sjogren's Syndrome
- Tendinitis
- Any hormonal imbalance
- Hypothyroid
- TMJ
- Abnormal hormonal levels (estrogen, progesterone, and cortisone) often accompany fibromyalgia. You may wish to consider being tested for these. They can all be treated very effectively with diet and/ or exercise as prescribed by your physician.

SO NOW, "WHAT IS FIBROMYALGIA?"

Your answer can be something like, "Fibromyalgia is an autoimmune disorder that causes pain, fatigue and stiffness throughout the body and makes me susceptible to health risks that most other people could easily fight off."

It can be difficult to describe this complex and mysterious illness without going into great detail (which the person who is asking does not want to hear). You can use this basic explanation, along with the information in this chapter, to form an answer that you, personally, feel comfortable with.

CHAPTER 2
WHAT CAUSES FIBROMYALGIA?

"There Are Possibly a Number of Factors Involved"

"What Fibromyalgia is" is a syndrome; what causes fibromyalgia remains a mystery, as there is no clear agreement amongst researchers as to its exact cause.

According to the National Institute of Arthritis and Musculoskeletal and Skin Diseases, "The causes of fibromyalgia are unknown, but there are probably a number of factors involved".

Many people associate the development of fibromyalgia with a physically or emotionally stressful or traumatic event, such as an automobile accident. Some connect it to repetitive injuries. Others link it to an illness.

People who have rheumatoid arthritis and other autoimmune diseases, such as lupus and Lyme disease, are particularly likely to develop fibromyalgia. For others, fibromyalgia may just seem to occur spontaneously.

While there is no clear agreement about what causes fibromyalgia, most researchers believe the fibromyalgia syndrome results not from a single event but from a combination of many physical and emotional stressors.

Below are just a few of the speculative causes of the fibromyalgia syndrome:

AUTOIMMUNE DISEASE

Fibromyalgia pain does not have any significant evidence to confirm it to be an inflammatory response, but its symptoms do resemble those of a rheumatic illness.

In an autoimmune disease, the immune system attacks the body's own healthy tissue, causing inflammation and tissue damage. The treatment that medical doctors use for this inflammatory condition is to suppress the immune response.

You will want to keep this in mind: although fibromyalgia is not an autoimmune disease, many persons who suffer from fibromyalgia also have associated autoimmune diseases which do cause inflammation.

IMPROPER BALANCE OF THE MICROBIAL TERRAIN

In my definitely "non-expert" opinion, this has more to do with fibromyalgia syndrome (and all other immune system disorders) than any other "cause". I do hope more research in this area will be forthcoming.

Our bodies house many types and number of microbial menagerie within the gut. Our immune system is what keeps these communities of bacteria in balance.

These bacteria, if in balance, keep our bodies humming along in a healthy state of being; but you want balance. If one community supersedes their appropriate amount allowed in the balanced state of being, then the result could be devastating.

Margaret McFall-Ngai, professor of Biology and Immunology at the University of Wisconsin, first proposed this theory. This hypothesis could have wide-ranging consequences for medicine. *See http://www.arizonaadvancedmedicine.com/articles/immune_syste m_dysfunction.html

By supplying our bodies with proper nutritional diets and supplements (such as probiotics, prebiotics, natural anti-inflammatories and antioxidants), we support our immune system so it can do its job of keeping things in balance.

TRAUMA

There are those who seem to develop fibromyalgia shortly after some sort of physical trauma such as an episode of flu-like symptoms, a car accident, or emotional trauma etc.; the list of causative factors can be extensive and varied.

UNDIAGNOSED HYPOTHYROIDISM

Dr. John C. Lowe, former Director of Research for the Fibromyalgia Research Foundation, and one of the nation's pioneers in the diagnosis and treatment of hypothyroidism, said this about fibromyalgia: "When I refer to fibromyalgia, I am referring to a certain set of symptoms and signs of too little thyroid hormone regulation of tissue."

According to Dr. Lowe, undiagnosed hypothyroidism is the causative factor for fibromyalgia.

EPSTEIN BARR SYNDROME

For a time, it was believed that fibromyalgia was caused solely from a serious flare-up of the Epstein Barr Virus. This caused many to fear that fibromyalgia was transmittable.

As it turns out, most people have been exposed to the Epstein Barr Virus by the time they are teenagers and get over it completely. The physical trauma that the Epstein Barr Virus causes to the body could conceivably motivate the domino effect that leads to Chronic Fatigue or Fibromyalgia in some people.

There are people, however, who get over the initial symptoms of Epstein Barr and then experience flare-ups that may compromise the immune system later on in life.

Therefore, yes; "Epstein Barr syndrome could affect fibromyalgia...just as anything that compromises the immune system could affect fibromyalgia"...but fibromyalgia is not transmittable.

NON-RESTORATIVE SLEEP

It would seem that some research is suggesting that the major concern here is sleep deprivation, but many believe sleep deprivation is not so much a cause as it is a problematic symptom.

When a person is diagnosed as having sleep deprivation, it does not necessarily mean that the person is not getting enough sleep, but that the sleep that they are getting is non-restorative sleep.

Throughout the day, as you use your muscles, there are little tears made in the muscles. These tears are restored as you sleep. There are many other kinds of repairs being made in the body during our restorative sleep periods such as hormones being produced etc. For some unknown reason, persons with fibromyalgia seem to have a problem with being able to go into this restorative stage of the sleep cycle.

Non-restorative sleep is when you awaken feeling tired and run-down even after a full night's sleep. This non-restorative sleep can, in time, lead to many problems throughout the body.

One very important occurrence happens during the restorative sleep period. As the body repairs itself, it also produces the brain chemicals needed for the body to work correctly. This effect on the brain chemicals, resulting from a lack of restorative sleep, is enough to cause a weakening of the immune system.

Some of the same effects commonly experienced in persons with fibromyalgia could be duplicated in a normal, healthy person if they were not permitted to sleep over a long period of time. The only difference being that after a good night's sleep, a healthy person's body will "bounce back" once they are permitted to sleep.

SLEEP APNEA

If your doctor suspects sleep apnea, he may order a sleep study. If the resulting diagnosis is sleep apnea, you may see a lessening in your symptoms and a subsequent reduction in the number of flare-ups you normally experience by treating this condition.

The only problem that may arise here is the very methods used to treat sleep apnea may prevent some light sleepers from being able to sleep. If this occurs, talk to the people in charge of the sleep lab about the problem; the solution may be as simple as trying a different type of sleep mask.

BRAIN CHEMICAL IMBALANCE

For some reason there seems to be a problem with brain chemical imbalance for those who have fibromyalgia.

The needed signal input from neurotransmitter brain chemicals, such as serotonin and dopamine, is not as readily available as needed (perhaps from lack of restorative sleep). Again, brain chemical imbalance may not be a cause so much as it is a reactive symptom.

These neurotransmitters send signals throughout the body that our bodies need to survive. For example, it is these transmitters that are responsible for our knowing to move away from a hot fire before we are burned.

If the same transmitters worked incorrectly, they could magnify pain signals to say that a larger amount of pain was being experienced than really was being experienced. They could report that a small rubber ball that hit your toe caused the same degree of pain that a hard baseball thrown at your toe would have caused.

It is not that you have low pain tolerance...it is your body magnifying the pain signals that you are receiving. If your body were unable to make these pain messages, you would feel absolutely no pain.

The pain you feel is real; it is there for your protection. This is what your body sends to tell you how things are and what needs your attention. Your body makes the pain, not the thing hitting you.

It would be the job of the chemicals serotonin and dopamine to correct that report before any "substance P" (P for pain) is released into the spinal cord (this "substance P" is what permits the body to transmit pain signals). So the body sends the serotonin and "natural brain opioids" (happy chemicals) to modify these pain signals.

Dr. Patrick Wood, a senior medical advisor to the National Fibromyalgia Association, put it this way: "Dopamine is a natural analgesic. So here you have a brain in which, when you hurt the individual, the pain reliever is not released."

I personally know a woman whose son has this problem in reverse. His brain does not perceive pain as it should either.

Why the pain messages do not get processed properly through to the brain is unknown. He has the sense of "touch" just as most anyone does, but his body does not seem, for whatever reason, to receive pain messages properly. He has no problem with going outside on a winter day when it is below freezing, wearing only a nylon t-shirt, shorts and sandals…though there may be 6 inches of snow on the ground. For some reason, he does not feel "the pain of being cold".

He also loves working with wood-shop tools, and when he occasionally injures himself, does not realize it. He thinks it amusing that his mom freaks out when she sees him bleeding.

He can "feel" the sensation of touch, but either his neurotransmitters do not work right or his body does not supply substance "P" as it should. For whatever reason, his body has feeling, but it does not perceive pain as it should.

Therefore, here is another example of what can happen when there is a problem with brain chemical imbalance.

LOW SEROTONIN LEVELS
In this search for a common cause, some have alluded to the fact that low serotonin levels are common in individuals with fibromyalgia; are low serotonin levels a cause or just a result of the cause?

You could over-simplify this by stating that the two major ingredients the body needs to produce this serotonin properly are sunlight and at least 7 hours of sleep.

A reduction of sunlight causes a decrease of serotonin available to the body. This is why you have some people beset with seasonal depression caused by limited amounts of sunlight in the winter months.

Likewise, non-restorative sleep diminishes serotonin action...so there is going to be a decrease in the amount of serotonin to your body. This decrease in serotonin puts you at a disadvantage when it comes to modifying pain signals.

Therefore, as I said earlier, this sounds very simple; "people with fibromyalgia simply need more sunshine and more restorative sleep, or just more serotonin".

If only it was that simple...brain chemistry, however, is much more complex than that and there is obviously a more sinister plot afoot.

Now, is the problem really that there is not enough serotonin? Perhaps the problem actually lies with the function of the serotonin receptors that enable the serotonin to do its many jobs.

On the other hand, maybe the problem is in the amount of substance "P" that the body produces in relation to the amount of serotonin.

And so on and on go the speculations into the complex study of the brain and its many functions. We can only hope science will eventually be able to unravel this baffling puzzle.

At this time, all you can do is treat the symptoms. No matter that there seems to be no known single cause; fibromyalgia sufferers all have the same symptoms in common.

As an analogy, imagine three people with migraine headaches. They all three have the same symptoms of a migraine headache in common (headache, nausea, light sensitivity etc.) but the trigger that caused these symptoms of migraine headache is not the same for all three people.

The cause of one person's headache may have been their exposure to certain allergens. Another person's headache was, perhaps, from stress. Finally, the third person may be having problems with their eyes. Three different things causing each person's migraine headache, yet they all have one thing in common; "they all three have migraine headaches".

This is the way it is with fibromyalgia. Whatever the cause or causes of fibromyalgia may be, the one thing all individuals with fibromyalgia have in common is that *"they all share the same basic symptoms"*.

So now we understand that fibromyalgia is a syndrome...and a syndrome is a collection of signs, symptoms and medical problems that tend to occur together but are not related to one specific cause.

CHAPTER 3
JUVENILE PRIMARY FIBROMYALGIA SYNDROME

Subtle Symptoms Are Often Misdiagnosed as "Growing Pains"

Because the occurrence of Juvenile Primary Fibromyalgia Syndrome (JPFS) in children and teenagers is increasing, diagnosing the disorder early is important.

Treatment involves support from the family and paying careful attention to the child's lifestyle. To increase the child's ability to function during this time when the symptoms are at their worst; special attention should be given to their sleep habits, exercise, diet and stress levels in order to decrease the fibromyalgia symptoms.

The majority of children seem to either outgrow their symptoms in time or learn to care for themselves in such a way that they will not aggravate the symptoms. However, this is a condition that seems to come and go throughout life; often being influenced by their present state of health.

By paying careful attention to a healthy lifestyle, young people with JPFS should have no problem leading very happy and successful lives.

Sometimes it is very difficult for parents to recognize a problem like fibromyalgia in children. Unless the symptoms come on suddenly and are so pronounced that the parents feel the need to seek medical help, it is likely to go undiagnosed.

Children, primarily teens, will often exhibit symptoms that parents do not notice because the children do not think of this as being an illness; they just think of it as being their fault that they are having these problems.

If they are experiencing any pain, the pain they feel is not a major pain like appendicitis or a sprained ankle would be. They may complain that their arm hurts or their leg hurts; and they may not even complain about it at all until asked to do something.

If the parent does check out the complaint, the first thing they would do, of course, is check for fever, swelling or inflammation. If there is no fever or visible cause for the complaint, the pain is explained away as "growing pains" or "you probably strained a muscle when you were playing". The child looks healthy, eats well, does not have a fever and there is apparently no swelling or inflammation.

The things a parent should be aware of are any changes from the child's normal behavior. However, if the changes are so subtle, the parent may not notice them unless the child says something.

Below are some symptoms that a child may exhibit:

- Changes in their sleep patterns
- Hard to get the child awake in the mornings
- Child may have trouble getting to sleep at night
- Child may be repeatedly late for school
- May have trouble with sleepiness during classes
- Excessive use of snacks to "keep awake" while doing their homework
- Excessive use of "sweet snacks" to keep their energy up
- Always tired and too easily labeled as "being lazy"
- Sudden drop in grades
- Trouble with school subjects that require more analytical processing
- Avoiding their friends
- Bouts of irritability

What I have just described is often accepted as "a normal phase of being a teenager". This is why JPFS so often goes undiagnosed. Only occasionally will a child mention the more obvious symptoms that alert the parents that something is wrong like:

- "I did badly on the test because I slept through the whole thing"
- "I feel so spaced out all of the time"
- "Some things do not seem real to me anymore"
- "I cannot stay awake in some of my classes"
- "I stopped eating lunch with my friends because I cannot stand the noisy cafeteria"

The majority of children seem to either outgrow their symptoms in time or learn to care for themselves in such a way that they will not aggravate the symptoms.

THE PARENT'S POINT OF VIEW

Do not be overly concerned if you did not immediately recognize these symptoms. Often the child does not realize that their problem is a health problem. This makes it very difficult for a parent to realize there is a problem unless the child confides in them about some of what they are experiencing.

JPFS seems to come and go throughout life; therefore it is extremely important to find a naturopathic doctor who specializes in treating such autoimmune dysfunctions as fibromyalgia. These children do not want to look forward to a lifetime of taking strong medications and living with their unhealthy side effects.

By paying careful attention to a healthy lifestyle and being aware of what things in their lives trigger negative responses in their bodies, people with JPFS should have no problem leading very happy and successful lives.

As a father, physician and nurse,

I have a special place in my heart

For children

And I know the brief window

Of opportunity we have to teach

Them simple lessons that can

Lead to a lifetime of

Good health.

Richard Cannona

****

CHAPTER 4
SEEKING MEDICAL HELP

"You should feel at ease with your doctor"

A Naturopathic Doctor who specializes in disorders of the immune system would be the ideal doctor for any illness arising from a diseased immune system, but such doctors are not always accessible. Some people have to travel a great distance in order to see such a doctor.

After a diagnosis has been made and treatment has been decided, arrangements are usually made for future long distance treatment.

If this is not an option for you, then it is essential that you choose a physician who is knowledgeable of fibromyalgia or willing to take time to learn about it and work with you in finding the best way to treat it.

If you are having trouble locating a doctor, you may be able to get some help online by contacting various fibromyalgia associations. Another resource could be your local Independent Living Center. It is very likely that they have members who have fibromyalgia, chronic fatigue, Lupus or MS who could aid you in finding doctors who are familiar with conditions of the immune system.

SELECTING A DOCTOR

You should feel at ease with your doctor. If your doctor makes you feel badly about yourself or does not listen to your concerns about the direction your treatment is going, then drop them immediately. You deserve to have a doctor who is dedicated to finding help for their patients.

Depending on what your individual needs are, your doctor should be prepared to recommend podiatrists, physical therapists, occupational therapists, massage therapists, various exercise programs etc. to help in your treatment.

I will always be grateful to the woman I met when doing some research. I had been to doctor after doctor for years trying to find answers to why I experienced this great exhaustion, recurring pain and so many other problems.

For the past year, I had been in such constant pain…it was unbelievable that something so devastating could happen so quickly for no apparent reason.

This lady had MS and recognized my problem to be an autoimmune problem and insisted I go to her "wonderful doctor" who had helped her so much.

Therefore, I went to this "wonderful doctor" with a list of everything that went wrong with me from the time I was 17 years old (when it seemed all my health problems suddenly began and my whole world changed). I also listed the results of all the tests that had been run and their results.

I was almost daring him to make sense out of this whole thing. He read my entire list and then carefully applied pressure to several spots here and there on my body and asked if it hurt…it definitely did…he then began to explain that from the information on this list and the extreme pain caused by simply applying pressure in these "pressire points", I had every indication of having an illness known as fibromyalgia; unfortunately there was no cure, but we could treat the symptoms.

It didn't matter so much that there was no cure because for once I had a name for the "beast" that had turned my life upside down.

FIRST MEETING WITH A PHYSICIAN

- On your initial visit to your doctor's office, take along a self-written symptoms information sheet.

On this information sheet, you need to make a note of when your problems started, what they were and all of the many symptoms for which you have been trying to find answers.

- Include information concerning all test results.

- Abnormal hormonal levels often accompany fibromyalgia, so you may wish to discuss with your doctor having tests run for:

  1. Estrogen levels
  2. Progesterone levels
  3. Cortisone levels

No hormone medications are needed to treat these kinds of abnormal hormonal levels...they can be treated very effectively with diet and/or exercise as prescribed by your physician.

TREATMENT

Once a diagnosis of fibromyalgia has been made, your physician will prescribe a pain medication that seems to work best for you. Not all people respond to the same medications, so it will take some experimenting to find the one that suits you.

The problem that follows the using of prescribed medication for fibromyalgia is that once your doctor prescribes one drug, you then must deal with not only your original symptoms, but also the new side effects from the drug.

Fortunately, medical science is waking up to the use of herbs as acceptable healing tools, especially in Europe.

Informed doctors, aware of the serious side effects of some of the drugs that they would have to prescribe for pain, recognize the danger in taking such drugs for an ongoing condition that may last for years.

It would be advisable to seek the advice of a nutritionist or naturopathic doctor about what natural supplements would be recommended instead of using prescribed medications that have known side effects.

As with even prescribed medications, not every person is going to respond in the same way. It may take some experimenting on behalf of the nutritionist or naturopathic doctor before finding the right combination of supplements that work best for you...but there truly are nutritional supplements that work just as well as, if not better than, prescribed medications.

Your doctor may also prescribe an antidepressant; this is not because he thinks you are depressed. There seems to be a link between low serotonin levels and fibromyalgia. Many antidepressants work by increasing your serotonin levels because it is a "happy hormone". Some physicians prescribe these mild antidepressants to their fibromyalgia patients hoping the increase of extra serotonin will help to reduce the pain signals.

There are natural supplements that are also used to promote higher serotonin levels. If you are not going to a naturopathic doctor you can talk to your nutritionist about what would be your safest resource.

Try to remember before each doctor's appointment, to make a list of any new symptoms about which you may be concerned. It is very important that these new symptoms not be passed off as part of fibromyalgia. It is true that fibromyalgia symptoms often "copy" the symptoms of more serious illnesses, but if these are new symptoms, they should not be taken for granted.

PODIATRIST

If you experience fibromyalgia pain in your feet, it can cause pain so severe that it makes each step you take feel like you must have several broken bones in your feet.

A visit to a podiatrist would be a very smart move if you have any pain in your feet. You will thank yourself for doing this later.

You should also mention any numb spots on the soles of your feet or tingling/vibrating sensations in your feet or legs to the podiatrist.

For people who have fibromyalgia, most podiatrists advise buying good quality shoes that support your feet well. They should have a supportive arch and a sole that provides both support and flexibility. Because of tendonitis often being a problem with fibromyalgia sufferers, you may need shoes that are made especially to meet these needs. Your podiatrist will guide you in the choice of shoes that meet your own special requirements.

Most podiatrists recommend walking, in moderation, as a good beginning exercise for individuals that have fibromyalgia...but you must start gently, wear supportive shoes and contact your doctor at the first sign of pain.

PHYSICAL THERAPIST

Before setting up an exercise program, you should consult your doctor about enlisting the guidance of a physical therapist. The therapist you choose must be knowledgeable of the limitations of fibromyalgia patients.

Even if you are not interested in setting up an exercise program at this time, a physical therapist can teach you various stretches that will keep your muscles from tightening up and becoming stiff, show you ways to accomplish such things as how to get out of bed more easily and ways to move your body to make life a little easier and less painful.

When I started going to a physical therapist, she could not understand why my body was so very stiff and sore, yet my legs were so limber...it didn't make sense. We finally realized it was from "stepping over baby gates".

With very small twins in the house, we had to make sure they could not gain access to certain rooms, such as the kitchen, unattended. It was much easier and quicker for me to carefully stretch my legs over a baby gate when going through the doorways than to constantly take the gate down to pass through.

"This little bit of daily stretching kept my legs limber enough that I could

drive and walk better."

Besides physical therapy, there are many other therapies also available for treating fibromyalgia (*see Coping with Fibromyalgia*).

OCCUPATIONAL THERAPIST

Fibromyalgia affects all areas of your life, so it is important to find ways to minimize the problems it causes.

An occupational therapist is a physical therapist that specializes in disabilities such as rheumatic disorders. They can be helpful in determining changes that need to be made in the way you sit and move in order to cause less stress to your muscles and lessen your pain. They help disabled patients to recover, and improve the skills needed for daily living and working.

An occupational therapist can be especially helpful if you choose to continue to work. They can evaluate your work situation and recommend changes in the way you go about your daily activities. They can guide you in the performance of all types of activities…ranging from using a computer to caring for daily needs such as dressing, cooking, eating, and driving.

They can customize an individual treatment program for you to make it easier for you to perform daily activities and do comprehensive home and job site evaluations to offer advice on how to prevent unnatural stretching, twisting or excessive bending down to gain access to regularly used items.

They can also recommend adaptive equipment, train you to use it and offer guidance to family members and caregivers.

NATUROPATHIC DOCTORS AND NUTRITIONISTS

Anyone with a chronic illness needs the correct supplements for supporting his or her individual needs. Without guidance, people with chronic illnesses can, out of desperation, become vulnerable to the many so called "miracle cures" for fibromyalgia.

A naturopathic doctor or nutritionist can recommend natural supplements for the problems for which you are seeking help. Their guidance will help you to:

- Prevent the wasting of your money on products that you actually do not need.

- Help you avoid using supplements that could possibly interact with other supplements that you presently take (natural does not mean it will not interact with other supplements, prescribed medications, or foods.).

- Assure you of getting the best products for your needs and the results you are looking for.

If a nutritionist is unavailable in your area, you may try looking online for local nutritionists or asking at various health stores, where nutritional supplements are sold, for a listing of nutritionists closest to your area. Be very cautious about taking the advice of a salesperson...they are not nutritionists.

Naturopathic practitioners in the United States can be divided into three categories. There are traditional naturopaths, naturopathic physicians and other health care providers that provide naturopathic services. Their main objective is preventive medicine.

Naturopathic doctors (NDs) have training in medical and clinical sciences (i.e. biochemistry, pharmacology, pathology etc.). In addition, they have extensive training in a full spectrum of natural medicines and therapies.

NDs spend more time with their patients to find the underlying causes of illness and to determine an integrative treatment plan...Do not be surprised if your first visit lasts for almost 2 hours...it sometimes takes that long to do a full evaluation of your physical problems.

Naturopaths can do blood chemistry tests and use other diagnostic tools as needed. They are trained in minor surgery and intern in clinics with doctors of many different specialties, but in California they cannot prescribe pharmaceutical drugs except for hormones.

Currently 16 states, 2 US territories and 4 Canadian provinces license naturopathic doctors. Each licensed state's scope of practice varies. For example, in Arizona, naturopathic doctors have equal standing with MDS and Dos/ they can prescribe medications and do diagnostic tests.

California had a license for naturopathic doctors until the 1950s when it was voted out. A new license began in 2004, with some limitations.

.

CHIROPRACTORS

Most chiropractors are also very knowledgeable about the use of herbs and supplements as well as stretches that are beneficial for fibromyalgia patients.

THE FIBROMYALGIA CHALLENGE

When life presents us with a challenge, we can triumph over this challenge in many ways.

- Accept that we are challenged

- Do not allow discouragement to let you give up hope

- Seek advice from others who have withstood the same challenges

- Search for blogs, groups and sites that offer positive support

- Seek out those who are best qualified to advise you

- Set goals…No matter how small the goals, each one attained is one step forward

- Lastly, offer hope and support to those enduring the same challenges that you have also endured.

~Alice Mowery Burnworth~

CHAPTER 5
COPING WITH FIBROMYALGIA

Therapies, Lifestyle Changes and Natural Alternatives

This chapter presents the many therapies and practices that fibromyalgia sufferers have used to reduce the impact of fibromyalgia on their lives, but just as with anything else that has to do with fibromyalgia, not every person responds to the same treatments.

PRESCRIBED MEDICATIONS

Physicians do the best they can by treating the different symptoms as they arise. One of their choices for pain treatment would most likely be SSRI's or SNRIs. These mild antidepressants are very helpful as they increase the serotonin to the brain, but they do have various side-effects and you should know what they are so you can make an informed decision about whether you actually want to use the medication or not.

.

You should research each new medication that your doctor prescribes. I cannot emphasize enough here just how important it is that you take an active interest in your treatment program.

Anytime your physician prescribes a new medication, you should get in the habit of looking up its "side-effects" online. There are sites available on the internet such as: webmd.com, eMedTV.com and drugs.com. These offer information about side effects and possible drug interactions on most all prescribed drugs and supplements.

Keep this in mind when researching "possible side-effects"; possible side effects means that "some" people have experienced these side effects and possibly more people will (maybe you?). You need to consider whether the side effects are minimal enough to not be concerned about. If you are concerned, then you need to talk to your doctor about using a different drug with less serious side effects.

NARCOTIC DRUGS

Some doctors prescribe narcotic drugs such as opiates for pain. I personally believe that narcotic drugs should never be given for chronic pain. (Chronic pain is pain that is going to be around for who knows how long versus pain from a serious injury that will only be around for a few months).

A person living with chronic pain, day after day, may be tempted to increase their dosage if there is an increase in their pain. This is a dangerous thing to do especially with narcotics such as opioids.

Narcotics are addictive. This means that when you first start taking them, they are great and really reach the pain. When they eventually no longer help you, your doctor raises the dosage. Again, they are great and really reach the pain. This little scene repeats itself several times until you are taking the maximum dosage.

When the max dosage no longer helps you, you will find yourself having to slowly withdraw from the use of a drug that no longer helps you anyways. At that time, your body will be demanding an increase, but by law the doctor will not be able to prescribe a higher dosage.

When I first started taking opiates, the effect was great; it really reached the pain. I found out later that the euphoric feeling that I felt when I first start taking this drug is caused by the limiting of oxygen to the brain. Eventually I found myself dependent on a drug that is known to kill brain cells. When I realized that I had become dependent on this drug, I was outright angry with myself for not recognizing the obvious signs.

You should be wary of any medication that seems to help you at first, but after a while the dosage repeatedly needs to be increased in order to get the same relief. This is the nature of a drug that is addictive. Run; do not walk, away from this drug.

For me, this goes back to when I was seventeen years old and had developed a peptic ulcer. My doctor prescribed phenobarbital to help with the healing process; not warning me of possible addiction. When it seemed the prescribed one tablet per dose was not helping as much, I started taking two; then eventually, ten months later, I was still on the drug and had just increased the dosage to four tablets.

It so happened that the father of a friend was a drug enforcement officer. When this friend saw me shaking uncontrollably because it was time for another dose of "medicine" he recognized the symptoms and sat me down and asked if I was on drugs. I denied it..."Of course not, the doctor prescribed this for my ulcer." This friend told me to get to a doctor and get off the stuff...he probably saved my life. Believe me, it was not easy and had it not been for another very good friend who helped me every step of the way (and whom later I married) it would have been even harder.

Getting back to opiates, they are not a comfortable drug to wean oneself off of, especially when you are dealing with pain versus the memory of the original euphoric pain relief provided by the drug. But I did gradually get off of it and was glad of it.

The US government and the FDA have issued warnings against these drugs. These opiates go under such names as hydrocodone, oxycodone, codeine, fentanyl, hydromorphone, meperidine, morphine, and tramadol (Ultram).

The American Society of Addiction Medicine says, "Drug overdose is the leading cause of accidental death in the US, with 47,055 deaths occurring in 2014; Opioid addiction is driving this epidemic, with 18,893 annual overdose deaths related to prescription pain relievers." That is 18,893 people in one year who actually died "accidentally" taking opiates. These people did not want to die...they were just people wanting to get away from pain.

Maybe some intentionally took more than their prescribed dose because they wanted extra pain relief, but maybe (because of the problem that people with fibromyalgia have involving short term memory and mental confusion) some simply forgot they had already taken it, accidentally took the highest dosage twice, overdosed on opiates and never woke up again...ever...regardless the reason; 18,893 people in one year died from taking prescription opiates!

Overdosing on prescribed medicine is a great concern; it happens too easily to people who are not aware of the outcome.

I was talking to a nurse about the overuse of prescribed pain relievers. She works in an emergency room trauma center. She said they see so many patients who come in after auto accidents; they have broken ribs, arms or legs and are in intense pain. But since these patients already have higher levels of prescription pain medication in their system than the emergency room nurses are permitted to give, they suffer greatly. She said it breaks her heart to see them suffer such unbelievable pain as they beg for something more powerful; all because their doctor chose to use powerful narcotics for "chronic pain relief". Narcotics should never be given for "chronic" pain.

You can find more information on opiates at:

www.pbs.org

www.ssn.org

www.deaddiversion.usdoj.gov/

MY PERSONAL EXPERIENCE WITH PRESCRIBED MEDICATIONS

After unsuccessfully trying to find a pain medication that would help me, my doctor prescribed a mild anti-depressant. This particular type of anti-depressant is found in a class of drugs known as "serotonin-norepinephrine reuptake inhibitors" (SNRIs). These drugs increase the serotonin and norepinephrine levels available to the brain cells. In many patients this has proven helpful in reducing pain.

After I started taking the mild anti-depressant, I could actually sit down and feel like "ah-h-h, it feels good to sit down", for the first time in almost a year. I still had chronic pain, but now when I sat down, I could feel a degree of "relief". Sure, because of the fibromyalgia pain, I still slept on two body pillows with three other pillows positioned wherever I needed them most and my sheets hurt me where they lay against my body, but now, I could feel my muscles relax when I lay down.

Before this, my body was so wracked with feverish pain that there was not a second that I was not in extreme pain. The pain was everywhere…in my neck, shoulders, arms, legs, feet, back and hips. There was no lessening of pain whether standing or sitting. There was no release of muscle tension…no feeling of "ah-h it feels good to sit down and rest".

My doctor was concerned because he could not find a pain medication that would relieve all the pain, but I assured him that he had helped more than he could imagine.

After prescribing several different pain medications that just "did not touch the pain", my physician eventually prescribed the opiate "Tramadol", I was hopeful because it was the first pain medication that ever came close to touching the pain…but at what cost?

Over time, my prescribed dosage of Tramadol was gradually increased until I was taking the maximum dosage. But when even the maximum dose eventually no longer helped, I did not appreciate finding myself in a state of "drug dependence" and having to wean myself off of the drug (not easy or fun, but do-able).

It took me five years to come to the realization that these daily medications were just going to have to stop. There was no way I could go through another five years of this. My daily routine was to take my medicines in the morning and then look forward to spending the entire morning until shortly after lunchtime, doubled over with upper and lower abdominal cramps and stomach pain.

Within a year, I was weaned off the prescribed medications. During this time of gradually weaning myself off prescribed medications, I proceeded to develop a treatment program using such things as pacing my activities, taking natural supplements, and developing a healthy diet. By the end of the year, I felt much better and in control of my life again.

Now I was learning how to "prevent" symptoms rather than just expecting medication to do it all. I still had fibromyalgia and still had flare-ups, but the pain and other symptoms were much less than when I was taking prescribed medications. I was learning to avoid those things that caused flare-ups by paying attention to how foods, activities etc. affected my body.

NATURAL ALTERNATIVES

The term "Natural Alternatives" does not refer to "Nutritional Supplements" only.

Natural Alternatives can refer to any number of therapies, supplements, diets, exercise programs, changes in daily routines…even small things such as setting priorities, pacing and adding laughter to the day. Anything that reduces symptoms and causes one to feel better without depending entirely on the use of prescribed medications is a Natural Alternative.

As with all alternative treatments, you should keep your doctor, pharmacist and nutritionist advised of any choices of treatment you decide to try before starting something new.

On the following pages, you will find brief descriptions of various therapies and other natural treatments that many people have allegedly used to help relieve fibromyalgia symptoms:

THERAPIES

ACUPRESSURE

Acupressure therapy is very similar to acupuncture, only it does not use needles to restore balance to the body. An Acupressure practitioner uses fingers, knuckles, palms, elbows or feet to apply pressure to specific areas on the body. This pressure is held for between 3 and 10 seconds.

Some people do acupressure on themselves. To do this, you simply locate the painful or tender spot and press with your fingertips or knuckles; then gradually increase the pressure for a few seconds or until the pain starts to ease up and you feel the muscles relax.

Some find it helpful to relieve painful spots on their backs by lying down on a tennis ball placed carefully on the painful area. The idea is to massage around the painful area by moving your back on the tennis ball until you locate the painful spot. You then hold it in that position until you feel the intense muscle pain ease up.

ACUPUNCTURE

Studies show that acupuncture may alter brain chemistry, causing a measurable release of endorphins (the body's natural opioids) into the bloodstream.

There are many styles of acupuncture, depending on where the practitioner studied.

- Chinese acupuncture requires the use of larger bore needles and a more aggressive needle action.
- Japanese acupuncture involves using thinner bore needles with a relatively gentle approach.

*besides the traditional approach to acupuncture, there is now the use of Electro acupuncture and Laser acupuncture.

There are precautions that you should take before you try acupuncture. You should first make sure the acupuncturist is licensed and very experienced in acupuncture. It is also very important that you make sure the acupuncturist uses only disposable needles.

BIOFEEDBACK (MIND-BODY TRAINING)

Licensed professionals such as psychologists, psychiatrists, dentists and physical therapists normally do biofeedback.

People with fibromyalgia often experience chronic pain in specific places on the neck, shoulders, back, hips, arms and legs when pressure is applied to them. Biofeedback operates on the theory that you can reduce these symptoms by directing your concentrated thought on a specific area of the body.

In biofeedback, a machine is used to measure electrical impulses coming from your body. You can learn how to affect a certain part of your body in a positive way by watching the machine's signals.

One of the more elementary training procedures may be something like concentrating on raising the temperature in one of your fingers.

By watching the machine's signals, you will learn what constitutes a positive effort and what does not…and you will become more attuned to your body's reactions to the impulses you are sending out.

- Electromyography (EMG) is the type most commonly used for fibromyalgia. It measures the electrical impulses coming from your muscles.

- Peripheral Skin Temperature (PST) measures electrical impulses given off from your blood flow. This could possibly be useful in warding off persistent cold or Reynaud's Phenomenon.

- Electroderm Response (EDR) is used for anxiety and depression, to monitor electrical impulse from sweating reflexes.

- Brainwave Electroencephalogram (EEG) is used for correcting all sorts of ailments including depression, sleep apnea and others.

- Breathing Biofeedback is used for relieving anxiety and fatigue…monitors your pulse rate and how fast you are able to breathe.

CHIROPRACTIC SESSIONS
Most chiropractors recommend a "full body alignment" because bones, muscles, joints, tendons and ligaments work together as a connected system, each dependent on the other to keep it functioning efficiently.

Some people prefer chiropractors who use Applied Kinesiology, but most chiropractors have different techniques and philosophies, so you still have to ask around and look until you find the one that is best for you.

Although many people attest to pain relief from chiropractic massage, you should talk with your doctor before starting treatments.

LUMEN PHOTON THERAPY
(Low Level Laser Therapy, Phototherapy or Near-infrared)
At this time, research has shown no adverse side effects from this form of therapy, but more research is needed in order to set definite dosages to be used and how often it should be used.

The many studies that have been done on low laser technology, to date, report reduction in pain and an increasingly longer time between painful episodes. Laser therapy is really a form of light therapy, and lasers are important because they are convenient sources of intense light at wavelengths that stimulate specific physiological functions.

MAGNET THERAPIES
Magnet therapy is the application of magnetic fields to the body. The force created by the negative/ positive poles of the magnetic fields is supposed to stimulate the body's cells and increase circulation (thus increasing the amount of oxygen to the tissues). This is to reduce inflammation and create overall better health.

1. STATIC MAGNETIC THERAPY
"Static" Magnetic Therapy is the type used by fibromyalgia and arthritis patients. With this form of magnetic therapy, patients purchase devices that can be attached or applied to the body such as: magnetic bracelets and jewelry, magnetic straps for wrists, ankles, knees and the back, shoe insole, mattresses, magnetic blankets (blankets with magnets woven into the material), magnetic creams, magnetic supplements, plasters/patches and water that has been "magnetized".

2. PULSED MAGNETIC THERAPY (ELECTROMAGNETIC COIL)
"Pulsed" Magnetic Therapy is a type of magnetic therapy (PEMFs) that is done in a clinical setting by a therapist or physician.
The intense electromagnetic pulses induce electrical signals at a subcellular level that stimulates chemicals in the cells to repair

damaged tissues like bone fractures.

PEMFT is widely accepted by the medical community for certain kinds of bone fracture repair and recent studies do indicate that using it for depression appears to be promising. Unfortunately, using it for pain management or wound healing has not been backed up with any accepted medical research as of yet.

MASSAGE THERAPY (VERY EFFECTIVE FOR FIBROMYALGIA)

Many people who have fibromyalgia insist that massage therapy is the most beneficial of any therapies they have used. You will need to find a therapist that is familiar with fibromyalgia.

You can seek the advice of your doctor or contact a local fibromyalgia group for a list of qualified massage therapists in your area. You can ask them how long they have been practicing and what techniques they use.

Massage therapy includes a variety of different techniques, such as stroking, kneading and palpating muscles. During massage, hot and cold therapies are often used to increase blood flow and to relax the muscles.

The types of massage therapies most often used for fibromyalgia are:

- **SWEDISH MASSAGE**…the form of massage most often used in North America. Its purpose is to increase oxygen to the muscles, thus flushing out toxins and making the muscles healthier and more flexible. In Swedish massage, the thumbs, fingertips and palms are used to stroke the body in long, gliding movements, along with kneading, tapping and vibration techniques.

- **DEEP TISSUE MASSAGE** targets the deeper layers of your muscles and tendons by using a more intense massage to loosen up hardened or inflexible muscle tissue and tendons, releasing chronic tension and pain. This does result in some pain immediately following treatments, but usually disappearing within a couple of days.

- **MYOFASCIAL RELEASE** targets the stiffness and tightness caused by myofascial pain. The thin layer of fascia tissue covering muscles and organs can tighten up and result in pain. By stretching these areas of tightness and holding the stretch, the fascia can relax and relieve the pain.

PACING (*MY GREATEST TURNING POINT*)

Though pacing may not essentially be a therapy, it is a therapy of another sort. My greatest turning point came when I started using pacing.

I was having an exceedingly bad flare-up. The pain was so relentless during this flare-up that all I wanted to do was lie down; but I could not just let myself lie there and waste an entire day when I had so much to do. I decided I would at least do some laundry and lie down during machine cycles. This way the day was not a complete waste of time and I could get the rest I desired. I spent the day repeating this idea of taking rest periods in between the laundry cycles.

I started by putting a smaller load of laundry into the washing machine than usual, so I would have less laundry to handle at one time and it would be easier to make the clothes look nice. Then I would lie down.

When the washer was through its cycles, I put the clothes into the dryer and put another wash into the washer. After turning the machines on, I would again lie down.

After folding away the small dryer load of clothes, I would lie down until the current wash load was through.

I repeated the procedure throughout the day until the laundry was completely finished. I not only accomplished a great day's work in spite of the painful flare-up, but also found a new way of doing things.

When I realized how well this "work/rest" idea worked, I decided to try the same work/rest idea with housework. This also worked well, so I started experimenting with work/rest periods on a daily basis. This was truly the turning point for me.

After a time, I was feeling stronger because I was able to be more active than before. The fibromyalgia symptoms were still with me, but I felt better about myself now and I felt more in control of my life.

This newfound hope gave me the courage to take control of my treatment program. I decided to spend the year gradually discontinuing all medications and using natural alternatives in their place.

I began to replace these prescribed drugs with natural supplements and in time, even the opiate was no longer a part of my life. (**Important note** it can be extremely dangerous to discontinue some medications without a physician's guidance. Keep your doctor advised of any changes you are considering in your treatment.)

After about a year of using pacing (as I found out later it was called) and using natural alternatives, I was finally able to keep the fibromyalgia symptoms more manageable than I had ever experienced with prescribed medications (and without the painful stomach and GI cramps).

REFLEXOLOGY (ZONE THERAPY)

Reflexology is a therapeutic technique in which pressure and massage are applied to specific spots on the feet and/or hands that match up to other places and organs throughout the body. The locations of pressure points on the foot are thought to mirror the placement of organs within the body.

Reflexology is not the same as standard massage therapy that concentrates on relieving pain and tension from muscles. Reflexology attempts to heal parts of the body, which cannot be touched from the outside by manipulating pressure points on the feet.

A treatment session usually lasts about half an hour. Because your reaction to the treatment can be unpredictable, allow for extra time after the session is over.

STRETCHING (TO INCREASE BODY FLEXIBILITY)

Not all forms of stretching are appropriate for persons with fibromyalgia.

*Do not start any type of stretching routines before discussing it with your doctor or therapist. *any program that requires the tensing of muscles should be started cautiously and under close supervision.*

Stretching should always be enjoyable, never rushed or painful. Always remember to "warm up" before you start and to breathe in deeply through your nose and breathe out through your mouth.

If you are going to start a stretching program, you may find it very beneficial to do the stretching in warm water as this is easier on the muscles. If you find it hard to hold a stretch, you may require assistance.

TYPES OF STRETCHING ROUTINES:

- **YOGA STRETCHES**: helps to restore flexibility and strength to your body and reduces stress levels

- **PASSIVE STRETCHING:** similar to the routines used at the beginning or end of aerobic exercise

- **ISOMETRIC STRETCHING:** increases strength and stamina of muscles. It involves the clenching and relaxing of muscles.

  Isometric stretching is easy to do and can be done at work and home.

- **ACTIVE STRETCHING**: First, you stretch and then hold that stretch for about 10 seconds. You use only muscle strength to hold the position...no assistance from hands.

  active stretching can be somewhat challenging for most people with fibromyalgia. But over time, you may develop a small degree of success in this type of stretching, resulting in an increase in muscle strength and flexibility.

- **DYNAMIC STRETCHING**: Dynamic stretching is not recommended for persons with fibromyalgia. It should only be done with caution and under the guidance of a professional therapist. Fibromyalgia is suspected of being a connective tissue disorder, so this type of stretching should be avoided in order to avoid damage to your joints.

It involves very slowly and very carefully stretching your body, allowing the target joint to reach its full range of motion, such as extending your leg out in front of you as far as it can go. You must not bounce or use quick movements in reaching your goal, as this could cause serious damage to your joints. This type of stretching is meant to be achieved over time…it must not be rushed.

**Do not use dynamic stretching if you suspect you may have a connective tissue disorder such as Ehler's Danlos (often referred to as flexibility syndrome or "double-jointedness").

TRIGGER POINT INJECTIONS

Trigger point injections are given in a physician's office by a medical specialist such as a physiatrist, neurologist, orthopedist or pain specialist.

Often, a nerve block will be injected to prevent the chance of pain. Perhaps the most common trigger point injection substance is a mixture of lidocaine and bupivacaine; this offers the benefits of immediate numbing action of lidocaine and the slower but longer lasting benefits of bupivacaine for pain relief.

Beware of a practitioner who wants to inject long-acting local anesthetics, or those that are highly concentrated, or the drug epinephrine as these can all cause muscle death.

EXERCISE
Why exercise when you are tired and in pain?

Autoimmune disorders are not caused by a lack of exercise and exercise will not cure them. But the problems associated with the lack of exercise will cause much more pain and debilitating fibromyalgia symptoms. This could be the difference between living a productive and active life and living a more painful, inactive life.

In order to reclaim or continue an active lifestyle, you will have to take on the challenge that fibromyalgia and many other autoimmune disorders present. No matter where you are, no matter how badly fibromyalgia has made you feel, you can get back on top; it just may take more time if your muscles are in an extremely inactive state.

When you have a debilitating illness or live with excessive pain, it is only natural *"to not want to move any more than you absolutely have to"*.

No one likes to be told they have to exercise, but when it comes to your muscles; the less you do, the less you can do.

If you have been extremely inactive, you would probably be best to think of it as a "movement program" rather than an exercise program at first.

Just doing something every thirty minutes or so (like walking over and picking up a magazine, getting a drink of water, walk around your desk, walk around your bed...anything to keep movement flowing throughout the day) is a very good way to start. Movement will prevent deconditioning and stiffness from setting in.

There is nothing wrong with starting an exercise program measured in seconds rather than minutes if you have been extremely sedentary. Even if you only exercise for sixty seconds per session, and do the sessions five or six times per day, you will actually be getting about five or six minutes of exercise per day; if you do them faithfully every day, you will benefit.

If simple repetitive motion bothers you, you may want to try holding the exercise position for several seconds instead of repeating it. This may take longer to see results, but will definitely help in the long run.

Sometimes the best way to start something new is to keep a journal so that you can see just how much you are actually progressing. This does not have to be in a book, even a small monthly planner book will work.

You could, on the date that you start exercising, jot down what you are doing now and a short sensible goal that you wish to achieve in two weeks' time. At the end of two weeks, you may or may not have achieved your goal, but it will encourage you when you see that you have improved since your starting date.

Deep breathing (from the lower part of the diaphragm) will help to relax you and it improves the circulation of oxygen in your body.

Stretches help with flexibility. The more flexible you are, the easier it will be to move with less pain.

Various good exercise programs involve simple stretching and very low impact exercises.

Some people, for example, use tai chi with good results. This is a method of using various slow stretches along with deep breathing.

If you are able to tolerate a more active type of activity, try resting three or four minutes for every minute of exercise. (*If your walk to the mailbox and back takes five minutes, then you could rest for about fifteen minutes as you read your mail.*)

If you have been inactive for so long that deconditioning has set in, you may not even be able to sit up in a chair. Follow your therapist's instructions very carefully. Your body will eventually begin to regain strength and you will be able to do more and more…but it is going to take patience and determination.

Remember that magnesium and malic acid are very important when exercising. Dr. Jacob Teitelbaum, wrote in the Fatigue to Fantastic Newsletter, "Magnesium and malic acid are also critical. When malic acid and the other compounds are low, the body often has to shift to the very inefficient *anaerobic* means of generating energy. This contributes to the abnormal buildup of lactic acid that occurs after exercise; causing muscle achiness and fatigue".

It is very advisable that you consult with your physician and with a therapist that is knowledgeable of fibromyalgia about your current physical condition before starting any exercise program. It is also important with any exercise program that you guard against falling if your muscles are in a weakened state.

EXERCISE ROUTINES

MIRANDA ESMONDE-WHITE (USING ESSENTRICS)

I discovered an exercise program that is so very helpful for flexibility; you can access some of the short sessions on youtube.com. These short sessions are by Miranda Esmonde-White. The great thing about her exercise program, using Essentrics techniques, is that you do not feel like you are exercising, you just feel like you have just had a relaxing stretch. She also has videos available on Amazon.

The one thing I like about her routine is that it is slow and relaxed; this is very important for anyone who has fibromyalgia. Whatever you use as your exercise routine, you do not want to jerk or move quickly; your muscles need slow movements so you will not suffer negative results. For a better understanding of the muscles of a person who has fibromyalgia read "The Collagen Connection" chapter.

AEROBIC EXERCISE

Aerobic exercise is any exercise that gets your blood circulating and increases the rate at which you breathe.

Just about any activity that gets your body moving can be considered aerobic. Simple daily aerobics could include walking, cycling or swimming. Therefore, this could be as simple as a brisk walk to your mailbox and back.

Before starting any exercise program, you should talk with your doctor or therapist.

If you are interested in using an aerobic exercise program for your exercise routine, consider only doing low impact aerobics if you have been very inactive and only with your doctor's permission.

- Aerobic exercise is good for your heart and strengthens your muscles so you are less apt to injure them.
- Aerobic exercise can actually decrease pain because it causes your body to release endorphins, which are natural painkillers.
- Aerobic exercise can often cause you to sleep better and stay asleep longer.

BALANCE EXERCISES

You will find many articles that provide helpful exercises for improving your balance and stability on ehow.com.

Just type in www.ehow.com and in the search box put "exercises for balance problems".
……………………………………………….

The Balance Manual…For exercises to improve stability and prevent falls. This manual starts out with extremely easy exercises and emails new exercises to you each week. The exercises are in video form and they are free.
www/thebalancemanual.com
…………………………………………..

Harvard University has written pamphlets on exercises to improve stability and prevent falls…these are a little pricey and many of the reviews say the pdf form is not as good as the pamphlets.

………………………………………………

MUSCULAR CONDITIONING/STRENGTH TRAINING

Recent studies performed by Harvard University have shown that a progressive regimen of strength training helps to reduce the symptoms of fibromyalgia.

STRENGTH TRAINING

Strength training without weights is popular with fibromyalgia sufferers because it targets all the major muscle groups of the body; you use the resistance of your own body instead of using weights. Your goal is to increase strength, endurance and muscle tone throughout the body so you can move about without so much pain…not to create bulging muscles.

WEIGHTLIFTING PROGRAMS

Many are set up in such a way that they let you choose one of several exercises for each of the nine muscle groups as your exercise. By doing these exercises without the use of weights you will have an exercise program that will let you actually achieve overall muscular development without overuse of any one muscle group.

When I first began, I did not use any weights with these exercises and I only did one exercise for each muscle group. I did not repeat any of the exercises, I would slowly do one exercise, hold the position and slowly release. This made for a very interesting stretching routine. I was surprised when I began to see good results within a week.

My son David developed Ankylosing Spondylitis when he was in his late teens. This is what some refer to as a "killer arthritis". This type of arthritis causes the body's joints to fuse together (even the ones in the chest that have to expand in order to breathe).

David was the one who recommended this program to me. David's condition had quickly worsened until finally his spine was fused and he could not turn his head to the side. His doctor could not believe how much the disease had progressed in one so young. He said most people do not reach his stage of the disease until they are in their 60s.

Now his knees were starting to swell enormously as they do before they begin to fuse. David had to get his doctor's very reluctant permission in order to join a gym. He went to the gym every single day except for weekends and, using weights, did the exercises in Bill Phillip's weight-lifting program.

Within a short time, he was seeing amazing results. Not only was he getting stronger, but he also lost weight and looked great. Then came the unexpected benefit...the arthritis went into remission. Occasionally he will have a flare-up, but he continues the exercises (less aggressively) and the flare-up regresses. *This is how important exercise is.*

You should consult your physician before starting any exercise program. Ask your doctor to recommend a physical therapist that understands how to help persons that have fibromyalgia.

If you feel an increase in fibromyalgia pain once you start an exercise program, you should notify your doctor and your therapist at once. The simplest exercises, done repetitiously, may cause fibromyalgia flare-ups. Some therapists, whose training did not include working with fibromyalgia patients and their special needs, can end up causing a lot of pain. (*Regrettably, I speak from experience*)

When you first start exercising, you may possibly "feel it "in your muscles a little, but you should definitely not feel it to the point that each session results in a flare-up that takes you a week to get over.

Exercises that strengthen your "inner-core "are usually very simple to do. These muscles help with your posture, and general well-being. They strengthen your deep inner muscles and improve the abdominal muscles, diaphragm etc. Ask your therapist about these exercises...

....
Exercises Programs for the Inner Core Muscles
American Council Exercise (AceFitness.org) you can search this site for free core-exercise programs... Very good instructions.

....

The Mayo Clinic has an excellent slideshow for exercises that are used for strengthening your inner core. Most of them are very easy to do and very effective. Do not "overdo" them because they look easy...you may regret it.

http://www.mayoclinic.org/healthy-living/fitness/multimedia/core-strength/sls-20076575?s=3
....

FELDENKRAIS (CONTROLLED BODY MOVEMENT TRAINING)
Awareness through movement lessons teach you the correct way to move with less strain on the body. Pain causes us to limit our movements and thus limits our lives.
Awareness through movement lessons are focused on how we move. The lessons begin with the idea that the correct way to move is the way that causes the least pain.

FOOD SENSITIVITIES
A well-nourished body is one of your best lines of defense when it comes to a compromised immune system, but some people with fibromyalgia find their symptoms worsen after eating certain foods. The most common offenders are dairy products, certain

preservatives, MSG and gluten. The best way to determine if you have food sensitivities is to pay attention to how various foods make you feel; this can vary from one person to the other.

If you suspect certain foods to be the cause of fatigue, indigestion or headaches etc. you could try keeping a journal for a couple of weeks. By recording your reactions after eating these foods, you may see a pattern forming after a couple of weeks. Possibly the best way to be absolutely sure a food is an offender would be to eliminate it from your diet for a period of time.

GLUTEN SENSITIVITY

The most obvious symptoms of gluten sensitivity are heartburn and general G.I. problems. The less obvious symptoms are inflammation, depression, brain fog, migraine headaches, joint pain and rashes.

If you have gluten intolerance or allergy, you will likely see a difference within a couple of weeks on the gluten-free diet. Many people who suffer with heartburn and G.I. problems will see a difference within as little as four or five days.

IMPORTANCE OF A GOOD NIGHT'S SLEEP

Addressing any sleep problems is the next on the list for management of fibromyalgia symptoms. Sufficient sleep is of key importance anytime your body encounters a stressful condition, especially if you have fibromyalgia.

With fibromyalgia there are the problems of achieving restorative sleep and of staying asleep once you fall asleep; for these reasons, allowing for adequate sleep time is of utmost importance. Pain and frequent insomnia are the main causes for not being able to stay asleep.

WHY IS MELATONIN IMPORTANT?

Your body produces melatonin to make you sleepy. Your body is programmed to start producing this melatonin when the amount of sunlight is diminished. This is so that in the evening, when it starts to get dark, you will wind down and get sleepy.

Modern day life compromises our body's natural programming. During the daytime, many of us find ourselves in an office with little or no sunlight.

This lack of sunlight causes the body to start producing melatonin. We, in turn, use coffee or soft drinks loaded with caffeine, to keep ourselves awake so we can do our jobs. Then we start craving sweet rolls of sorts because the caffeine messes with our insulin production.

When you go home in the evening, you find yourself exposed to bright lights from the TV, computer screens or any number of other gadgets that are backlit; it is like staring into a lightbulb. This suppresses your body's production of melatonin and makes it hard to get sleepy.

In order to get your body back in sync with a normal daily schedule, so you can sleep at night, there are several things you can do:

- Increase your exposure to light during the day

- Remove your sunglasses when safe to do so

- Try to find things you can do outside during the daylight hours such as taking a walk, take breaks outside or in a sunlit area, exercise in a sunlit area, study outside, have lunch on the patio or on a park bench.

- Open the curtains or blinds and let more light into your home or workplace. If you are working at a desk, sit as close to a window as possible.

- A light therapy box can be used to simulate sunshine. You can even find lights that program the amount of light they produce, according to the time of day. These can be especially useful during short winter days when there is limited daylight.

INCREASING MELATONIN PRODUCTION AT NIGHTTIME

- Turn off your television and computer a couple of hours

before bedtime. If your favorite TV shows are on later in the evening, just record them and watch them the next day, but earlier.

- Many people use the television to fall asleep or relax at the end of the day, and this is a mistake. Not only does the light suppress melatonin production, but television will actually stimulate the mind, rather than relax it.

- Do not read from backlit devices for up to an hour before bedtime.

- Use softer lighting in your home.

- Be sure the room you sleep in is dark or use a sleep mask to cover your eyes.

- Rather than turn on a lamp during the night if you wake up to use the bathroom, use a small flashlight; this will make it easier to go back to sleep.

- Keep the temperature in the room where you sleep slightly on the cool side, but not extremely warm or cool.

- If you cannot avoid or eliminate noise from traffic, barking dogs, loud neighbors, city traffic or other people in your household, there are several ways to block it. These include white noise machines, soothing music, running a fan (or an air purifier).

Our brains are constantly active throughout our sleep period; they do not just zone out. You could compare the brain to your computer in this instance.

Much like when you put your computer on disk cleanup, the brain takes in so much input during the day and it has to catalog these things in order to get the unimportant things filed into unimportant data folders that make room for important things. Then the important things will have to go into proper files etc. In the end, you end up with a less cluttered brain so you will be ready for a new day when you arise.

This is where we will draw the line between our brain and the computer. Our brain is in constant communication with our body; it does not actually "sleep".

Your brain is busy helping your body to produce all the things needed to actually produce growth hormones, which results in tissue repair and healing.

Your body has such incredible abilities to repair itself as long as it is supplied with the proper resources to work with, such as:

- A diet rich in vitamins, amino acids, oils etc. that your body can actually use to repair itself.

- Exercise (even very light exercise), in order to increase the delivery of oxygenated blood to your working muscles (remember, your heart is a muscle also).

- Proper hydration... Our bodies are 90% water and must have water for washing out poisons etc. and making needed repairs.

- Proper sleep routines are essential for our bodies to make the restorative repairs needed daily.

WHAT IS "PROPER SLEEP" AND WHY IS IT SO IMPORTANT ?

There are five stages of sleep and they usually repeat themselves about every 90 minutes.

The sequence of these five stages is not necessarily in order, and most of them, except for the deeper sleep stages, can be interrupted easily by outside stimuli such as noise, light or touch.

These lighter stages of sleep are important because they lead to the deeper stages; therefore, you need to do all you possibly can to prevent these lighter stages of sleep from being disrupted. Every stage of sleep is important, but body repair is usually associated with the deeper stages of sleep.

How to Help Your Body Prepare for Sound Sleep

- Set a regular bedtime and stick with it.

- You have to listen to your body for signs of being tired. This will help you to find the time your body is ready for sleep when setting up a sleep routine.

- Wake up at the same time every day.

- If you get to bed late, do not try to make up for it by sleeping in the next day. Get up at your regular time and stay up for two or three hours. You can then take a long morning nap to help make up for the lost sleep; this will make you feel better, but is not going to promote restorative sleep like a good night of sleep will.

- If you find yourself getting drowsy after dinner, find something to keep yourself active until the desire for a nap passes.

- If you want to change your bedtime to an earlier time, do it in 15 minute increments. Wait at least two or three days before going to another 15 minutes earlier. This will prevent 15 minutes of not being able to go to sleep due to the change in routine.

- Regular daytime naps can be a very positive thing, but they should not exceed one hour of total time allowed. Naps should not be taken after dinner time, or they could make it hard to sleep at your regular bedtime.

It is of key importance, for your health, that you do all you can to provide a good sleep environment. Some of the best ways to do this are to:

- Make sure the room temperature is at a comfortable setting.

- Use something like a body pillow or several well-placed pillows to relieve painful areas.

- Make sure the sleeping area is dark, quiet and conducive to sleep. If this is not possible, you may want to consider earplugs or a sleep mask (one that blocks out all light).

- Earplugs are not necessarily a safe solution for some people; other options could be "white noise machines", soft soothing music or running a small fan in the room for the gentle humming sound etc.

Before using even natural herbal sleep preparations, it is always important to consult your nutritionist and your pharmacist in order to determine if there could be a chance of drug interaction. *I have personally found that taking an easily absorbed magnesium supplement an hour or so before bedtime helps to promote sleep.*

One way of starting a good sleep program without using sleep inducing preparations is to eliminate long naps during the day. If you feel you need a nap, set a timer for 15 to 30 minutes.

This amount of time is sufficient to give you the rest that you want, but not long enough to let stiffness and pain settle in nor would this keep you from being sleepy at bedtime. If you take several naps during the day, the total time for one entire day should not equal more than one hour; any longer could interfere with a good night's sleep.

In place of napping during the day, sometimes you may find it equally restful to do something you enjoy such as listening to music or sitting outside on a nice day. Under normal circumstances, it would be advisable to limit this restful time or nap to no longer than 30 minutes (set your timer) before getting up and walking around. This will help to prevent painful stiffness.

NUTRITIONAL SUPPLEMENTS

Many people choose to use prescribed medications for fibromyalgia pain at first; however, as fibromyalgia symptoms could last for many years, most people gradually begin to look elsewhere for "long-term" relief rather than continuing with potentially harmful drugs over an extended period of years.

There are natural supplements that provide the same relief as the prescribed medications. But just as with prescribed medications, what helps one person may not help another. You will have to work closely with your nutritionist or naturopathic doctor in order to find what supplements are right for you.

Whether you choose to use prescribed medications for fibromyalgia symptoms or choose to use natural means (or a little of both) is a personal choice, but you should keep your physician, therapist and your nutritionist aware of any changes you make.

Because of the many deficiencies often associated with fibromyalgia, larger doses of some nutrients may be prescribed. For this reason, you may have noticed that some daily vitamin/mineral preparations are formulated especially for people with fibromyalgia. One such multivitamin is made in the form of a drink mix made by "Integrative Therapeutics".

Before embarking on a natural supplement program, it cannot be emphasized often enough just how important it is for you to see a certified nutritionist or a naturopathic doctor (ND) before you start using supplements for health problems. Each person is an individual, and as such, should be treated as an individual.

You will meet people who insist that what "cures" one person of fibromyalgia will cure all persons with fibromyalgia, but you can just chalk it up to their eagerness to help and their ignorance of the mysterious nature of fibromyalgia.

There are many therapies, nutritional supplements, dietary changes etc. that "help" help you cope with fibromyalgia symptoms to the point that you feel really great most of the time... But these are not "cures".

As you continue with those changes that have proven helpful in controlling your symptoms such as: pacing, stress management, natural supplements, dietary changes and therapies, you will continue to benefit from these lifestyle changes.

ASSOCIATED ILLNESSES

Most fibromyalgia sufferers have a myriad of associated illnesses and these should be addressed if you are to find to help you deserve. This is one reason why your Naturopathic doctor and nutritionist should know about your overall health before starting any kind of treatment program.

There may be health related problems responsible for your persistent frequent flare-ups. Health problems such as the ones listed below usually respond to treatment using nutritional supplements, and various therapies; thus giving you additional relief from the severity of your fibromyalgia symptoms:

- IBS
- Candida
- Adrenal exhaustion
- Hypoglycemia
- Stress-related problems
- Digestive problems
- Heart health
- Circulatory system health
- Kidney function
- Liver function
- Gallbladder problems
- Asthma

Besides including your health history, you may wish to make out a list of any health concerns you wish to discuss, such as the ones mentioned below:

- Low energy levels
- Problem falling asleep or staying asleep
- Strengthening the immune system
- Muscle tenderness

- Soreness after exercise
- Deficiencies that often accompany fibromyalgia
- Ways of increasing serotonin levels
- Improving sluggish memory
- Natural antibiotics and steroids
- Natural muscle relaxers
- Natural pain relief

Natural supplements should be taken with understanding and can be just as effective as many prescribed drugs, but you can easily waste your time and money needlessly by taking "this or that" supplement that is touted as the latest "cure – all".

You are a complex individual and you need someone who understands just how natural supplements can interact with each other or even counteract each other's effectiveness. Keep in mind also, that just because something is natural does not mean it is safe for you or that you can take it with no concern about the supplements, foods or prescribed medications that you take with it.

Any time you come upon something new that is supposed to help with fibromyalgia, check the Internet for any possible side effects that could affect any other health problems you have. Then consult your Naturopathic doctor or nutritionist before trying the supplement.

As you research fibromyalgia and familiarize yourself with the various supplements etc. recommended to treat fibromyalgia, be careful that your sources are reliable. Pay close attention to the Internet address of the site before you even click on it; you can usually tell if it is a reputable site.

There are many blogs that provide helpful advice from others who suffer with fibromyalgia and the information you glean from such sites will help to educate you on the role that nutritional supplements and therapies play in fibromyalgia related problems.

However, any advice should be backed up with quotes from reliable sources and your Naturopathic doctor or nutritionist should be consulted before you decide to try anything new.

Whether you decide to try the natural route completely or to use prescribed medications along with some natural alternatives, keep these three things in mind:

1. If there are no naturopathic doctors in your area, make an appointment with a nutritionist and let them guide you in determining what supplements you should use and what brands are the best sources. You will be more apt to find what you need, and you will likely save yourself a lot of money in the end.

2. If you are going to use natural supplements along with prescribed medications, be sure you clear all supplements with your nutritionist as well as with your doctor and pharmacist.

3. No prescribed medications, natural supplements nor any kinds of exercises or therapies are going to really give you the relief you want if you do not make the necessary adjustments in your attitude toward taking care of yourself and recognizing your limitations.

Practice good sleeping habits and "pace yourself" in your daily routines. Once you give your body the rest that it needs throughout the day by using pacing, and it gets the sleep it needs at night, you will stand a better chance of seeing a big difference in your body's response to treatment.

Some natural supplements, just like some medications, do not always make a big difference right away. This does not mean that they are not helping you in your battle against fibromyalgia.

Certain supplements will provide immediate help while others require a longer period to see their effects. This is something you will want to discuss with your nutritionist.

To Sum up my own experience with pain relievers versus natural alternatives

At the onset of fibromyalgia pain, I frantically needed pain relief. For five years, I depended on prescribed medication to give me the much-needed relief I needed. Yet even though it helped, no medication could get rid of all the pain...and the side effects from some of the medications followed me for years after discontinuing the medications.

Today I still have fibromyalgia, I still have inopportune flare-ups (but fewer than I did when I was on prescribed medication) and I have also been diagnosed with rheumatoid arthritis, but I feel in control of my life and I do not have to be concerned about the nasty side effects that come with prescribed medications. I know that I have to put a lot of preparation and effort into planning for things that another person may just take for granted, but it is worth it.

By applying lifestyle changes such as: pacing, getting sufficient sleep, and seeking out natural alternatives in place of the prescribed drugs, I found pain relief comparable to... No, make that much "better than" what I experienced with prescribed medication.

Let food be thy medicine

And medicine be thy food.

Hippocrates

****

"The six best doctors anywhere

And no one can deny it

Are sunshine, water, and air

Exercise and diet.

These six will gladly you attend

If only you are willing

Your mind they'll ease

Your will they'll mend

And charge you not a shilling,"

Wayne Fields

****

CHAPTER 6
MUSCLE SORENESS AND FATIGUE

What causes the soreness, fatigue and heavy feeling in your muscles?

Oxygen and nutrients for the muscle cells are carried through the bloodstream to the mitochondria, powerful little batteries that gives energy to the muscle cell. Muscle cells have many mitochondria and the more energy a muscle needs, the more mitochondria it will have.

Muscles love to be exercised; causing your body to send a regular supply of oxygen and nutrients to the muscles; keeping them healthy.

"Aerobic" Energy

The type of energy produced when the muscle's mitochondria pick up the oxygen and nutrients needed from the bloodstream for continuous repair and rebuilding of the mitochondria is called aerobic energy. Using this aerobic energy the mitochondria then sends into the muscles:

- Nutrients needed to do necessary repairs to the muscle,
- Energy needed for the muscle to contract and release
- Antioxidants to wash such things as lactic acid and waste products out of the muscle.

"Anaerobic" Energy

When there is a lack of nutrients being supplied to the muscles, there is another way for energy to be supplied, but this way is very inefficient and causes a buildup of lactic acid in the muscle (which causes pain). This is referred to the "anaerobic" process of supplying energy to the muscle and this energy comes from sugar.

When an athlete has been running for a long period of time, they will recognize this change from aerobic energy to anaerobic energy as a signal that it's time to stop and take a break. This short break gives the body time to catch up so the blood flow can, once again, efficiently supply the nutrients and oxygen needed by the muscles. The athlete will feel their energy returning again and know they can now continue with the run.

When there is a lack of needed nutrients being supplied to the muscles, the muscles cannot be receiving their energy from the aerobic source as before and will switch to anaerobic energy

The muscles cannot work as efficiently using the anaerobic energy source and pushing yourself to go on instead of resting will cause the muscles to not be able to wash the lactic acid and waste products out; resulting in pain and exhaustion. This inefficient energy supply is bad for the muscle in many ways.

Without the oxygen and nutrients needed to repair the mitochondria and the muscle, the muscle will eventually become covered with scar tissue (which causes pain) and the mitochondria (the power factory for the muscle) cannot be repaired properly.

Now this brings us to the reason why people with fibromyalgia suffer so much muscle pain and what they can do to help prevent this problem.

CAUSES OF FIBROMYALGIA MUSCLE PAIN

The Parker Institute's Department of Rheumatology and the Danish national Library of science and medicine in Copenhagen Denmark did a study of fibromyalgia patients and found them to have significantly lower amounts of intramuscular collagen protein in their bodies than the average person.

When a person exercises, their muscles are subjected to a kind of injury and the body then uses collagen to repair the injury to the muscles in order to make them stronger than before; putting the body in a constant state of repairing itself.

Since people who have fibromyalgia have significantly lower amounts of intramuscular collagen protein, it takes a longer time to repair these micro injuries, making the repeated use of a muscle result in pain and soreness.

In this same study they also found a defect that showed fibromyalgia patients do not experience a normal increase in blood flow when the patient becomes more active.

The cause of this lack of blood flow increase is to believed by many to be from conditions such as poor antioxidant status, poor thyroid or adrenal hormonal control, improper protein function or a lack of much needed nutrients such as:

- Vitamin B3,
- D-ribose,
- Co-Q10,
- PQQ,
- Acetyl l-carnitine,
- Lysine,
- Antioxidants such as vitamin E and vitamin C
- Magnesium/malic acid

This lack of extra blood flow makes it take much longer for their muscles to relax and recover than an average person's would
.

Therefore, if a person with fibromyalgia does not pace themselves by taking frequent rest periods when they are active, preferably before they are tired, they will find themselves stuck in this painful, anaerobic situation.

If the body is using anaerobic energy, there will be a buildup of lactic acid resulting in muscle damage and a breaking down of the collagen that holds the cells together.

This is why it is so important for fibromyalgia sufferers to avoid this anaerobic state by resting "before" they are tired and to not use an exercise program that is based on repetitive muscle action.

With this in mind, it is easy to understand why that although it is important that you exercise to keep your muscles healthy and to keep them from atrophying, it is also important that you exercise or move in ways that will not increase demands on the muscles. Using such repetitive movements can cause undue stress in the body's muscle groups, resulting in a flare-up.

Most therapists recommend that you use only low impact, non-repetitive types of exercise programs that are geared to your specific energy levels at this time. Your muscles will become stronger with time and your exercise routine can be adjusted according to your capabilities.

Moderate exercise is good because it not only keeps your muscles healthy, but it also makes it easier to move without putting unneeded stress on the body.

Many experts agree that "good old-fashioned walking" is one of the easiest and least stressful forms of exercise.

- Researchers at Indiana University found that five minutes of walking is enough to reverse the harmful effects to the arteries in the legs caused by an hour of sitting…

- Walking increases circulation and supplies more blood and oxygen to the muscles and organs.

- Walking regularly has been linked to improved memory and increased growth of new neurons.

Therefore, it stands to reason that a short walk could do an enormous amount of good without putting in a lot of stress on the body.

Discuss with your doctor or therapist just what kind of exercise program would be right for you.

THE COLLAGEN CONNECTION

How to Increase the Amount of Usable Collagen in Your Body

Up to 30 percent of all protein in the body is collagen and up to 70 percent of all the protein in the connective tissues is composed of collagen.

It is an essential ingredient in the makeup of ligaments, tendons, cartilage, bone and skin. Therefore, when your body becomes depleted in the amino acids needed to produce collagen, the muscles cannot be repaired adequately and activity is accompanied by acute pain.

As the body's natural ability to repair connective tissue and maintain hydration of cells diminishes, protein is needed to produce the collagen. However, most protein supplements do not contain enough raw materials needed by the body to produce this collagen.

The main builders of collagen that can be added to the diet consist of vitamin C (ascorbic acid), lysine, proline and distilled MSM.

Vitamin C is required to connect the two amino acids together (proline and lysine) to form collagen fibers.

Sulfur nutrients like MSM and bioflavonoids such as grapeseed naturally support these bonds, helping to maintain the natural strength and flexibility of collagen. Hyaluronic acid then is the flexible goo that fills In between the collagen strands.

If you wish to supply these collagen building materials by adding them to your diet, there are some very tasty ideas listed below.

SIMPLE SOURCE OF PROTEIN, LYSINE, PROLINE AND VITAMIN C

Whey protein isolate drink mixes can be a good source of protein in the diet. Choose a brand that does not have sugar or a load of additives in the ingredients. (Do not mix these in a blender as this could break up the beneficial properties.)

If you prefer to buy L-Lysine as a supplement, look for L-lysine in the capsule form rather than the pill form. L-lysine in the pill form is usually large and rough; the texture is like taking a pill made from cement.

VITAMIN C

One medium orange… contains 69.7 mg of vitamin C
Guava…1 cup contains 376.7 mg of vitamin C
Kiwi… 1 cup, sliced, contains 166.9 mg vitamin C
Broccoli… 1 cup serving contains 132 mg of vitamin C
Red bell pepper… ½ cup, chopped, contains 95 mg vitamin C
Papaya… 1 cup serving contains 88.3 mg of vitamin C
Strawberries… 1 cup contains 84.7 mg of vitamin C
Kale… 1 cup serving contains 80.4 mg of vitamin C
Green bell pepper… ½ cup, chopped, contains 60 mg vitamin C

MSM

There is a minimal amount of MSM in corn and raw tomatoes.
MSM, in the supplement form, may use one of two methods of purification.

- Distillation
- Crystallization

If you buy MSM supplements, be sure that they contain "Distilled" MSM. Supplements made using the Crystallization process may have "harmful impurities".

Distilled MSM is a form of sulfur found naturally in the body. One thing to remember is that MSM needs to be replenished throughout the day; so the supplement form should be taken 2 to 3 times daily.

As with anything that brings about natural healing, it will take time for your body to heal and renew and some people may see a difference earlier than others.

CHAPTER 7
THE CANDIDA CONNECTION

Candida Albicans can be a very real problem for anyone who has a compromised immune system.

Candida Albicans, a very real problem for anyone with a compromised immune system, is a yeast inhabiting our digestive system that normally does little harm as long as it is kept in check by beneficial microorganisms (the "good" bacteria).

The *good bacteria* help keep the Candida in check so that they do not turn into their fungal form and grow out of control, producing infections throughout the body. Such things as antibiotics, oral contraceptives, corticosteroid treatment, radiation treatment, prescription medications, daily stresses or bad diet choices such as sugar and highly refined carbohydrates can destroy these good bacteria.

If for some reason, the good bacteria are destroyed, the yeast then have the uncanny ability to change from their yeast form into a mycelial fungal form. Once the Candida is in their fungal form, they no longer can be controlled; they must be killed.

When you become physically or emotionally stressed, your body releases more of a hormone called cortisol. This hormone (cortisol) can weaken the immune system, and at the same time, cause elevated levels of blood sugar.

Since yeast feed off of sugar, elevated blood sugar levels can cause the yeast to grow much more quickly than normal.

There are only two ways to kill the fungal form and these are through diet and prescribed antifungal medication.

The problem with the medication is that many people cannot tolerate it and many others see no effects at all.

This uncanny ability of Candida to change from the yeast form into a mycelial fungus form makes it much harder to get rid of the Candida in the fungal form than it was to control them in the yeast form. When these fungi spread outside of the digestive tract they can lead to problems with our nervous system as well as our immune system.

Candida infection can hide in various parts of the body...around organs, the digestive tract or countless other body tissues. It can, in some instances, even become life-threatening.

For those with a chronic illness, it is so important that we stay on top of this problem at all times.

If you are already having a problem with Candida, you will likely notice an increase in your fibromyalgia or chronic fatigue symptoms.

EFFECTIVE TREATMENT
There are many treatments and supplements used to treat Candida, but the most effective long-term way to treat Candida is through diet.

Doctors can prescribe antifungals, but it is up to us to get our digestive tract back on the right track and support our immune system or the problem will crop up again and again... Putting our body in a state of constant bad health.

CANDIDA CLEANSING DIET
Unfortunately, the two weeks (or more) that you are on the strict diet are necessary in order to cleanse your body not only of the

infestation, but to cleanse your body of all the debris from the battle.

Drink a sufficient amount of water (8 to 10 glasses per day). These fungi emit toxins into your system and you need to do all you can to keep everything "flowing along" to wash them out or you are going to feel very sick…and your gut will have a harder time accomplishing its goal of cleaning house for you.

You may experience a day or so of loose bowel movements, but that is not to suggest that you are eating too much fiber; it could just mean that this is a part of the house cleaning project at hand. Taking a probiotic is necessary to increase the good guys in your gut… They are the ones doing all the work for you.

The simple, strict Candida diet is usually followed for a period of at least two weeks (some people find it necessary to stay on the strict diet a little longer before seeing results).

SIMPLE ANTI-CANDIDA RULES THAT APPLY DURING THE CLEANSING DIET AND BEYOND:

- Drink plenty of water

- Eat enough fiber to keep things moving through

- Take a good probiotic

- Drink Pau D' Arco tea once or twice a day… Hot or cold (antifungal and a mild tasting tea).

- Add up to 3 tablespoons of organic virgin coconut oil into your diet per day; a delicious addition to any hot foods or cereals, and excellent for stir frying.

- Sweeten foods with Stevia

- Drink ¼ cup aloe vera juice (not gel) every day. Aloe Vera juice (aloe water) improves the healing of any damaged areas of the intestinal walls and is thought to have some antifungal action. Drinking more than the ¼ cup per day can irritate the intestines. (I highly recommend George's Aloe Water; it tastes just like water, no bitterness at all)

- Mix 1 tablespoon organic raw apple cider vinegar (the kind with the "mother" in it) with 1 cup water and some Stevia for sweetening either before or after lunch and dinner. As an antifungal and antibacterial, the apple cider vinegar will help flush out toxins, mucous, and all types of harmful bacteria.

- For itchy skin problems caused by Candida (such as in skin folds and vaginal area), you can make a soothing topical preparation. Mix ½ cup aloe vera gel with 1 tablespoon warm (not hot) coconut oil. Whip the coconut oil into the aloe vera gel. You can add a small amount of vitamin E as a preservative. *Be sure the aloe has no ingredients other than pure aloe vera gel and possibly vitamin E which is often used as a preservative. Apply topically, as needed.*

THE STRICT CANDIDA CLEANSING DIET: (1 TO 2 WEEKS)

- Drink 8 to 10 glasses of water daily (80 ounces)
- Take a good probiotic daily
- Eliminate all forms of sugars
- Eliminate fruit and fruit sugars
- Eliminate milk and dairy products
- Eliminate simple carbohydrates (white flour, breads, pasta etc.)
- Eliminate nuts and nut butters
- Add lots of green, leafy and low-carb vegetables (no salad dressings except 1 tablespoon raw apple cider vinegar and Stevia mixed with 2 tablespoons water per day)
- Add healthy portions of meats (with no added sauces or breading)
- Add up
- to three tablespoons organic virgin coconut oil daily.

Once the strict diet is over, it is necessary to continue with the very liberal maintenance diet.

The maintenance diet is not so much a diet as it should become a "way of living".

MAINTENANCE DIET (EASY TO FOLLOW CANDIDA MAINTENANCE DIET)

Now that your two weeks of the strict diet is over, it is time to wage the "Cold War". You will notice that there are about as many variations of the strict Candida diet as there are people writing them. The real head scratcher here is that they all seem to sound right. They all seem to have very good reasons for their conclusions about what is and what is not acceptable.

However, the maintenance diet should not be that hard to incorporate into your daily life. It may be a little more time-consuming than buying "ready-made", greasy, sugary foods laden with additives and food enhancers that you can just toss into the oven, set the timer and walk away from.

One thing you want to consider when starting the maintenance diet; there is no one-size-fits-all solution when it comes to a healing diet because every person is different in their biological makeup.

Following a maintenance diet is actually as simple as establishing a more responsible attitude when it comes to what goes into your body. The choices you make will decide whether your immune system receives what it needs to continue taking care of your health.

The following suggestions will help you to work out your own maintenance diet. Using the guidelines below, try to develop a diet that is balanced, enjoyable and easy to stick with; the main idea is to keep your gut healthy and it will keep you healthy.

- Do not consider your selection of meat for dinner to be the main focus of the meal. Make low glycemic vegetable dishes the highlight of your meals.

- Cooked or raw, vegetables in their original form are the best choice as they are less apt to have unsafe oils, additives or preservatives in them.

- If you are having pasta and a large salad for dinner, use a pasta that is whole-grain and gluten-free such as ones made from brown rice, quinoa, or amaranth.
- For an exciting way to beef up a pasta dish, try adding a variety of freshly steamed vegetables into the pasta just before serving.

- Make salads more interesting as well as tasty by adding a large variety of vegetables into the salad.

- Nuts are great in a salad or just for snacks; just be careful to avoid the nuts, such as peanuts and pistachio nuts, that are closely associated with mold problems. Freshly shelled nuts are less apt to have a mold problem than pre-shelled ones sold in packages.

http://www.livestrong.com/article/440632-which-nuts-are-allowed-on-the-candida-diet/

- Top salads off with a dressing of vinegar, olive oil, Stevia, Italian seasoning and water, well shaken. You can get creative and add spices of your choice.

- For a creamier salad dressing, start out with some kefir and add sweetener and/or seasonings to taste.

- Another great creamy dressing can be made by whipping plain yogurt until smooth. Add water (1 tablespoon at a time) until it is the consistency you like. Now add sweetener and/or seasonings to taste.

- The more simple the meal, the easier it is to keep it anti-Candida healthy yet delicious. Vegetables that have a higher glycemic index do not have to be eliminated; just do not pair them with other high glycemic foods in the same meal and do not have them often.

- If preparing a recipe that calls for flour, use gluten-free, complex carbohydrate flours. You may have to add a little more baking powder because some flours are heavier. Add some xanthan gum to make ingredients hold together better and not crumble (1/4 teaspoon xanthan gum to 1 cup flour). Adding an egg can sometimes help the finished product to "stick together" better also.

- Try incorporating some nut flours along with your flour mixture... Such as almond flour or coconut flour (coconut flour will require a larger amount of liquids than other flours).

- Quinoa (keen wah), flour or flakes, is actually from a seed rather than a grain. It is tasty, gluten-free, high in protein, fiber and minerals.

http://authoritynutrition.com/11-proven-benefits-of-quinoa/

- Use only healthy oils such as virgin olive oil or virgin coconut oil.

- Do not eliminate fruits from your diet; just limit portions and choose low glycemic fruits such as ripened apples, blueberries or raspberries.

http://lowcarbdiets.about.com/od/whattoeat/a/whatfruit.htm

- Stay away from processed meats, cold cuts and deli meats. Even the most "innocent" looking ones have sugars, unhealthy oils and preservatives added.

- There are enough additives, sugars, coverings, MSG, taste enhancers, chemicals etc. in those processed meats to overwork even the healthiest person's gut as it tries to run interference for these toxic loads.

- If you do not have a problem with your blood sugar such as hypoglycemia or diabetes, and do wish to add natural sugars to your diet occasionally, choose the ones that are least apt to cause a problem. "Raw honey", "pure molasses" or "pure maple syrup" are natural sugars but these should not be eaten in excess of the suggested individual serving size.

- Avoid milks that are not fermented. Usable milks are those that are fermented (such as Kefir) or have cultures and probiotics added (such as most yogurts and some cottage cheeses). These can be very beneficial and should be a part of the diet.

- Almond milk is a very good substitute for dairy milk. It is best to use the almond milk that has no sugar added.

- For people with lactose intolerance, a yogurt-like drink called Kefir could allow them to add dairy into their diet again without side effects.

http://www.webmd.com/allergies/news/20030530/kefir-helps-lactose-intolerance

- Fermented vegetables such as fermented sauerkraut are extremely beneficial to the gut. The use of such fermented products is an excellent choice of prebiotics for your diet (most people prefer the benefits of fermented products that are *unpasteurized*). If you are concerned with the sodium content; note that some taste no better than others but have twice the amount of sodium.

As you work with this diet, you will begin to see just how easy it is to follow on a daily basis. It is very easily adaptable for dining out and holiday choice recipes also.

~Be good to your gut and it will take care of you~

CHAPTER 8
CONNECTING THE DOTS

Many times reactions are caused by the little things that go by unnoticed

When you live with a life-changing illness such as fibromyalgia, it is easy to be so caught up in daily struggles that you miss the obvious. By keeping a type of daily Fibro-Journal, you will be able to observe cause and effects more easily.

Many Software Programs, Apps etc. have a "Diary" that is set up in such a way that could be very adaptable for use as your Fibro Journal. Use whatever is best for you and "user-friendly" enough that you will be more apt to keep it up to date, because it is so important for you to do this.

NOT A PERSONAL JOURNAL
A personal journal is for recording events, sorting out your feelings or as a record of a spiritual journey. Although a personal journal can be a very therapeutic tool; you should do this kind of journaling in a separate book for saving and rereading for years to come.

When something is bothering you, it is helpful to find a way to let it go. The best way to do this is to write it down. Writing it out in something like a personal journal helps your mind to put the problem into perspective; and eventually let it go. Some people carry this a little further. They write what is bothering them down on a paper, wad the paper up and throw it into a garbage can.

The result of letting go is all that matters… and writing a journal like this may be just what you need as you deal with issues that accompany such an illness as fibromyalgia.

Nevertheless, this is not what a "Fibro-Journal" is all about. A Fibro-Journal is divided into four sections:

1. Daily Checklist
2. Flare-up Record
3. Treatments Used
4. Being Prepared

(SECTION 1) DAILY CHECKLIST

The Fibro-Journal's daily checklist is a brief ongoing record of each day's experiences concerning such things as: weather, hours of sleep, naps through the day, new symptoms, exercise (how active you were this day), new supplements or medications etc. In this checklist you will add anything that, on a daily basis, may affect fibromyalgia symptoms.

You will want to include a Notes section at the end of each day's list; this is for anything that you think worth mentioning, but is not listed on your daily checklist. These can be things such as: any changes, social interactions, annoyances, confrontations, personal telephone conversations etc.

By recording this information, you may see a pattern forming. In time, this vital information could reveal "flare up triggers" that otherwise, may have gone unnoticed.

Just as headaches and allergic reactions are triggered by foods, the environment, and stress, there are also triggers that cause fibromyalgia flare-ups. Some of these triggers, such as weather changes, are unavoidable; whereas some can be avoided if you know what they are.

Over time, your journal checklist may reveal many patterns developing that could show a link between what occurred several days ago and that flare-up you are experiencing today. At any rate, the fact is that once you start "connecting the dots", you will find it easier to avoid at least some of the things that trigger flare-ups.

Perhaps it is because we are going through so much when dealing with the symptoms, that we do not notice these patterns developing. Then again, maybe it is because it is hard to wrap your brain around the idea that anything so simple in your daily life could actually cause you to have an increase in symptoms.

As you begin to recognize some of your flare up triggers, you will notice some triggers are more evident, like a day of gardening or yard work, and sometimes the cause can be more subtle: such as a simple repetitive movement, PMS, not pacing yourself properly, lack of restful sleep or stress (good or bad) etc.

(SECTION 2) FLARE-UP RECORD

Though you are daily subjected to the pain associated with fibromyalgia, there are times, unfortunately, that people find themselves experiencing a worsening of symptoms (flare-ups).

In a section of your journal set aside for flare-ups you can record:

- Date of this present flare-up
- What your symptoms seem to be
- What you think may have triggered this flare-up
- How you are treating the symptoms
- What treatments, prescribed or natural, that you seem to be responding to well

(SECTION 3) FLARE-UP TREATMENTS USED

It is all too easy to forget what helped you the last time you had a flare-up when you are beset with the problems accompanying your present flare-up. If you have a place in your journal for recording what helped during the past flare-ups, this will be a great help to you.

This recording of symptoms, treatments etc. may be helpful to look back over when you are having another flare-up. This is definitely not the time to realize you have been negligent about keeping your journal updated.

(SECTION 4) BEING PREPARED

life goes on even though flare-ups may make it much more complicated. At home, being prepared may be as simple as having foods in the freezer that will make meal planning less of a chore.

Another helpful addition may be a good supply of disposable cups, plates, flatware etc. because sometimes even a dishwasher may prove to be more than you feel up to dealing with. You will want to prepare meals that use the least amount of dishes in preparation. A good example of this would be meals that can be baked in the oven using aluminum foil and/or parchment paper.

So keep a list of foods and supplies that you should have on hand to make meal time less of a hassle.

Keep the supplies up to date because you may not feel like going shopping during a full-blown flare-up.

If you have smaller children at home, keep a list of friends, relatives, or babysitters who would be willing to help during these times by taking turns coming into your home for a couple of hours and caring for the children while you take a rest and maybe popping a ready-made dinner into the oven for your family.

If you do have need of asking for help with children during a flare-up, you should also keep an updated list of information about those who have volunteered to help you such as:

- Any hours or days, that may be convenient or inconvenient for some helpers
- In what way certain helpers agreed to give their aid
- To prevent future problems, keep a reminder of problems that you may have encountered at other times in order to not repeat the same at this time.

POSSIBLE PREDICTABLE CAUSES OF FLARE-UPS

There are so many causes of flare-ups, and some are more predictable than others. As your notes and charts start pointing to the repeated appearance of certain activities etc. as possible reasons for future flare-ups, you will have a better idea of what to watch for.

Eventually you will see many patterns starting to form. This will help you to see, more efficiently, just what triggers your flare-ups. Now you can decide if there is some way that you can avoid these triggers or at least prepare ahead of time to greatly reduce their impact on you.

If the trigger is from doing too much at one time, then make a point of resting before you are tired; spreading work out over days or weeks instead of pushing to get it done at one time. If the trigger is stress, then make a habit of taking "mental breaks" by getting your mind off whatever is causing the stress. Give your mind something positive to think on and become absorbed in.

A mental break should be something that is a "mind absorbing" distraction such as reading a favorite book, engaging in some sort of artistic outlet or doing some kind of "mind games" such as cryptograms, Sudoku etc.

You may also find it helpful to use preapproved herbal stress relieving teas when you take a break.

WEATHER

Though you cannot change the weather, it does help when you know ahead of time how certain weather conditions usually affect you. You may be able to make plans more efficiently by taking into account the different weather that is normally associated with certain seasons.

Many people with fibromyalgia are so sensitive to weather changes that they will see increases in pain even before a change is detected on weather maps. These can be changes in air pressure, temperature, wind, moisture etc.

Some people will see a worsening of symptoms as the seasons become cooler and gradually a lessening as the seasons become warmer again. This does not necessarily mean that people living in dryer, warmer regions will have no fibromyalgia pain, but possibly they will not have as many weather-related flare-ups.

LUNAR CYCLES

We cannot overlook the many reports from people who do claim to be witness to the effect of the moon on people's behavior and body functions.

There have been more and more accounts of people with fibromyalgia saying they definitely see an increase in their pain during the full phase of the moon.

Professor Cajochen of the University of Basel in Switzerland, and his colleagues presented the first reliable evidence that a lunar rhythm can modulate sleep structure in humans.

Using stringently controlled laboratory conditions, Cajochen said, "The lunar cycle seems to influence human sleep, even when one does not "see" the Moon and is not aware of the actual moon phase".

In this study, Professor Cajochen proved that the lunar cycle modulates human sleep and melatonin rhythms. He proved that impaired melatonin production leads to complaints of nonrestorative sleep, and is increasingly recognized as being linked to insomnia complaints.

Fibromyalgia and chronic fatigue syndrome are also associated with impaired melatonin production and "nonrestorative sleep". The one thing that will definitely cause an increase in symptoms is an interruption in proper sleep.

Therefore, you may want to take note of whether the moon cycles affect your symptoms. Many people have indicated that two days before and two days after a full moon (and sometimes even a new moon) they see an increase in fibromyalgia and chronic fatigue symptoms.

I must admit that when I first heard this allegation, I thought it very laughable as I related the concept to my husband. It was only a short time later that I noticed an increase in my own symptoms. This was one of those flare-ups that occurs occasionally and does not seem to have an obvious trigger.

My husband, listening to me trying to make sense of this latest increase in symptoms said, rather matter-of-factly, "There is a full moon tomorrow".

I scoffed at the idea and forgot about it until the same episode replayed itself a month later and again my husband pointed out that there was a full moon in a day or so.

Well, after a few months of this, I finally had to concede that there truly was something to this as far as my body was concerned.

This does not necessarily mean that every full moon will cause an increase in symptoms, but for me, it happens often enough that I try to remember to be prepared by not making plans for social activities at that particular time.

I have even noticed that there are times that I see some increase in symptoms at the time of the "new moon" also, but not usually as pronounced as at the time of the full moon.

CHEMICALS AND ALLERGENS

Quite often the use of household cleaning supplies can trigger a flare-up, this is why it is preferable to use natural cleaning supplies such as white vinegar (an excellent antibacterial cleaner) for housecleaning when possible.

EXAMPLE OF A DAILY CHECKLIST:

Weather_____

Hours of sleep last night_____

Quality of sleep_____

Changes in medicine or supplements

_____

New exercise_____

Daily checklist continued

Total exercise time _____

Increase in symptoms_____

New symptoms_____

Activity level_____
Stress_____

Social life_____

Worries_____

Changes in routine_____

Diet changes_____

Telephone usage_____

NOTES_____

_____

CHAPTER 9
HELP! I'M HAVING A FLARE-UP!

Flare-ups can be so unpredictable and often seem to come at the worst of times

When flare-ups occur, the natural reaction is desperation. You are suddenly in so much pain and nothing you normally do is helping.

This is is no one definite answer for this dilemma known as a flare up, but that does not mean there is not any help to be had.

During this time, you need to pamper yourself by giving your body all the rest it desires and being careful to follow a few guidelines to avoid things that would delay your recovery:

❖ **A GOOD NIGHT'S SLEEP** during regular bedtime hours is essential for recovery...If you notice that you are not sleepy at bedtime, it may be that you are getting too much sleep during the day. You may be able to remedy this by replacing daytime naps with many periods of relaxation instead. It is also suggested that the length of daytime naps not add up to more than one hour total if you are having trouble sleeping at your regular bedtime.

❖ **GOOD NUTRITION IS ANOTHER ESSENTIAL** for your body during this time. Your body needs nutritious foods and supplements in order to repair itself. Try to eat a healthy diet.

Giving in to comfort foods will not give your body the support it needs at this time and could cause more complications.

Nutritious meals do not have to be time-consuming to prepare; they can be nutritious and simple. There are some examples of easily prepared, yet nutritious meals at the end of this chapter.

- ❖ **GET LOTS OF SUNSHINE** and a good night's sleep. Your neurotransmitters are overreacting and they need all the help that they can get; sunshine and good sleep habits are two important resources for such help.

Weather permitting, a short walk or just sitting in the sunshine for a short while is helpful. Some people find that "light boxes" made for the purpose of supplying different spectrums of light, are very beneficial at times when there is no sunshine in the forecast. *Do not use a lightbox within 2 to 3 hours of your regular bedtime.

- ❖ **PACE YOUR ACTIVITIES**… Pacing is especially important during this time. If there are things that you must attend to, try to sandwich these responsibilities between more restful activities.

- ❖ **PAMPER YOUR BODY AND MIND:** If you are at home it is easier to take care of flare-ups. If you have to work, try taking short five minute breaks as often as you can throughout the day. Totally relax during these break times. If this is not practical, try periods of just sitting down, closing your eyes, doing deep breathing, and relax your body all over even if only for a minute or two. Make this entire time of recovery as much of a pampered event as possible.

- ❖ **KEEP EVERYTHING AS SIMPLE AS POSSIBLE.** Keeping things simple can apply to any and everything in your daily life.

An example of keeping things simple could be to not complicate your life by taking on commitments that you may be unable to fulfill. When people ask you to commit to help or volunteer your time, you could begin by making them aware that, because your symptoms are so unpredictable, you can only work in positions that will not cause a problem if you had to call and cancel at the last minute.

You could also explain that you have to be careful to not be standing or sitting down for long periods of time as too much of either of these could cause an increase in your symptoms.
Many times it is best to just volunteer to assist those who already have assigned tasks.

In the workplace, keeping things simple during a flare up could involve putting off anything that is complicated or stressful until a better time.

At home, you could keep things simple by doing only very light housework rather than what you would normally do and planning more simple meals than usual.

* **AVOID STRESSFUL SITUATIONS** as much as in your power to do so. It often helps to let the people that you work with know that you are having a flare up and what you have to do or avoid in order to get better.

The flare up itself may last for several days to several weeks or even months (depending on what triggered it and how you handle it). How you handle this is up to you; just make sure that you get the rest that your body says it needs. Pamper yourself with warm (not extremely warm not extremely cool) baths or showers; do things that relax you and try to increase your hours of sleep at your regular bedtime.

* **TAKE NOTE ABOUT WHAT YOU CONSIDER RELAXING.**
When you are having flare-ups, you may want to be selective about the types of television programs and movies you watch. These should always be something on the "upbeat".

For a short time, you may want to consider not watching or perhaps recording for a later time, the type of movies that keep you on the edge of your seat: such as soap operas, tearjerkers or anything that arouses negative or anxious emotions. You will likely do best to find those things that have a more positive and non-stressful input. You can always record the movies or TV shows that are more apt to encourage such anxious emotions for later.

❖ CHECK YOUR DAILY JOURNAL NOTES

In the chapter "Connecting the Dots", you should find a list of things that would be most helpful to have on hand during a full-blown flare up. If you do not have these things on hand, perhaps you could give the list to someone to pick the items up for you.

Check your journal notes on what helped you the most when you had previous flare-ups.

In your journal, you could have a prepared "support team list". If you have small children, call your support team for help if you feel you need it. Support teams are usually friends, relatives and babysitters, who know you may be calling them for help occasionally. Just having someone with you, even for a few hours, that can watch the kids and maybe toss a ready-made quick meal into the oven for your family, can be a big help. (I am so thankful for the help of my mother-in-law and father-in-law.)

❖ EXPLORE POSSIBLE CAUSES

Look through your journal. Is there any record of changes in weather, activities, foods, health, sleep patterns or stress (physical and emotional) etc. that match activities preceding this flare up? If so, make a note of it in your journal.

Sometimes you can account for the flare-ups in this way and sometimes the cause is just hard to pin down.

You should have a place in the back of your journal set aside for recording flare-ups. You will want to include the date, present weather, activities etc. Over time, you may see a pattern developing that may be helpful in determining the causes of some flare-ups and make it easier to avoid future ones.

Keep an ongoing account of the flare-up and the way you are dealing with the symptoms. This information may be very important in dealing with future episodes.

Such things as yeast infections (Candida), unstable blood sugar levels, or increased uric acid levels can sometimes provoke flare-ups or at least complicate them.

If you suspect you may have one of these disorders, try to make the proper adjustments in your diet needed to stabilize the problem. You can try any of the tips below and see if they make a difference in the length or severity of the flare-up.

As you start your own diary of actions that help or do not help, you will eventually find yourself having more control over those things that influence your symptoms and possibly complicate existing flare-ups.

❖ CANDIDA DIETARY CHANGES

If you suspect yeast infection or overgrowth to be the cause of this flare-up these suggestions may help:

- Include yogurts that contain live cultures in your daily diet.

- Speak to your doctor and nutritionist about the use of an antifungal supplement (such as Pau D' Arco or Olive leaf extract).

- Depending on your individual needs, sometimes going on a gluten-free diet or an alkaline diet helps.

- Limit carbohydrates to complex carbohydrates only. Highly processed carbs are easy to grab and are found in most "comfort foods", but could cause Candida symptoms to worsen thus making the fibromyalgia symptoms worse.

- Make your meals as healthy and balanced as you can manage.

- Avoid sugars, refined carbohydrates (such as white bread) or anything else that is known to "feed" yeast growth.

- Include any supplements that help fight candida (vitamin C, B vitamins, Probiotics, garlic etc.).

▪ Take probiotic supplements 20 minutes before breakfast, and again before dinner. If there is a Candida Problem, you may need to continue taking this twice daily for several months.

▪ Speak to your nutritionist about supplements that can be used to correct any blood sugar problems (and sugar cravings).

❖ SIMPLIFYING MEALS

Make a list of meals that you can prepare in just a few short steps. You do not have to use expensive frozen prepared meals (that are usually packed with unwanted fats, sugars, sodium etc.).

Anything that can be "popped" into the oven to cook is great because "no cleanup"; just roll up the aluminum foil and/or parchment paper and toss it.

HANDY DISPOSABLE BAKING SUPPLIES:

• For broiling foods, you can line the pan with aluminum foil and spray with nonstick spray for easy cleanup.

• For regular baking purposes, you can use parchment paper over top of aluminum foil for healthier cooking. **Do not use parchment paper near the broiler element or for foods that will need to Brown.

• Parchment paper is great for microwave cooking. You can use it to either line your dish with or cook with by using it to wrap potatoes, chicken or vegetables in before placing inside the microwave.

• If you like the ease of tossing a plastic bag of vegetables into the microwave (steamables) you can save on the expense as well as avoiding the questionable plastic bag by putting the amount of veggies you want to cook onto a sheet of parchment paper; wrap the parchment paper around the veggies; turn upside down onto a paper plate and place it into the microwave (or if using a conventional oven, place on a baking sheet) and follow the cooking directions.

- There are various kinds of bakeware that have aluminum foil on the outside and parchment on the inside. These come in various sizes and shapes such as cookie sheets, loaf pans and cake pans.

- Another baking plus is aluminum foil lined with parchment paper. You simply turn the pan you wish to use for baking upside down; place the parchment lined foil over the pan (parchment side against pan) and press to shape. Turn the pan up right and place the foil lined parchment inside the pan (parchment side up).

- Paper bowls make great cooking pans for in the microwave (uncovered); just line them with parchment paper before adding the food. You can cook anything from rice to egg omelets in them. A word of warning, some of the cheaper brands of paper products are not made well enough to cook foods that have liquid in them.

- For crockpot liners: the most common "plastic-like" Crock-Pot liners are made from heat-resistant nylon resins. There are a few studies about the migration of chemicals from nylon resin liners to food, but at the current time there are no health risk warnings associated with these. Personally, I would rather use a parchment lined pan in the oven than take a chance on these crock- pot liners; but that is just my opinion.

YOU CAN PREPARE MANY EASY TO FIX FOODS WHEN YOU DO NOT FEEL LIKE FIXING A BIG MEAL:

QUICK MEAL EXAMPLES:

➤ **OVEN BAKED HAMBURGERS** You can purchase Low-fat hamburger patties, separated with parchment papers that can be stored in the freezer. Just slightly thaw them for about an hour; you can quickly pop the patties apart and put them into the oven for a quick meal (freeze the buns also, so you always have them on hand). Add a salad and your meal is ready.

➤ **ROTISSERIE CHICKEN** You can buy precooked rotisserie chicken at most supermarkets. Just add a salad (prewashed) and/or any other vegetables you choose for a quick meal.
When you buy precooked rotisserie chicken, buy two and put one in the freezer for later (Cut the chicken into smaller portions before freezing). You can prepare a quick meal using the frozen chicken, by simply reheating the chicken and serving with vegetables of your choice or by making it into sandwiches.

➤ **BAKED CHICKEN DINNER** Line a pan (foil covered with parchment paper). Place desired number of pieces of chicken onto the baking pan. Cover or surround with Chopped potato chunks (peeled or unpeeled) and vegetables of your choice.

Lightly cover entire pan with foil. Bake at 450° until chicken is well done and vegetables are tender(usually about an hour...depending on oven used).

➤ **FRIED ONIONS/PEPPERS OVER LEFT-OVER MEATS** Line a small pan with foil and spray with nonstick cooking spray. Add fresh or frozen chopped onions and/or sweet peppers.
Place in the oven on an upper shelf under the broiler; broil, stirring occasionally as needed. Watch carefully so they do not burn.
Remove the pan from the broiler. Pile the onions and peppers over warmed leftover meats and serve with prewashed salad greens or place the leftover meat, onions, peppers and prewashed salad greens on buns to make great sandwiches.

➤ **MINUTE STEAKS** Minute steaks... Season and broil in the oven for steak sandwiches. Add a salad of prewashed salad greens, onion and tomato for a quick meal.

➤ **PRE-SEASONED MEATS** (fresh or frozen) can be purchased by the number of servings you need. They are oven ready... Follow instructions for cooking. You can now choose your side dishes and your meal is ready.

➤ **ROSEMARY CHICKEN AND VEGGIES** (one serving)
Place one large sheet of parchment paper on large plate. Add one piece of frozen chicken breast.
Lightly spray chicken with no stick pan spray; add a sprinkle of rosemary and a dash of pepper.
Surround with a large handful of frozen veggies of your choice; add three tablespoons water.
Bake in microwave on high for five minutes; turn chicken over and bake until no longer pink.

If you wish to do this in the oven, lay the parchment paper on a sheet of aluminum foil.
Prepare food as directed, but add 4 tablespoons water. Pinch foil tightly shut and bake at 450 degrees for 45 minutes to an hour.

➤ **OVEN-BAKED BEEF STEW**
Using frozen or fresh stew meat chunks (prewashed and drained): Place stew meat in the center of a baking pan lined with aluminum foil/parchment paper.

Wash unpeeled potatoes and cut into quarters or generous-sized chunks. Place potato chunks evenly around the meat in the pan; cover the meat and potatoes with frozen sliced onions and peppers and top with any frozen or fresh vegetable mixture of your choice.

Season or add sauces of your choice. If you do not use a sauce, or the sauce you use is thick, add a few tablespoons of water. Cover with foil and let the oven do the work. Bake at 450° until potatoes and meats are done (usually about an hour, depending on your individual oven).

If you wish for the meat and vegetables to be lightly browned, remove the foil about 15 minutes prior to end of baking time. *Do not place under a broiler if using parchment paper.*

❖ **PREPARING VEGETARIAN MEALS**

➤ **PASTA** If you use whole-grain or gluten-free protein pasta, you do not necessarily have to add meat to the pasta for protein. Most whole-grain pastas have between 4 to 6 g protein per serving. All you have to add to the meal would be something like a prewashed side salad and pasta sauce.

If you want extra protein, you can always make a Greek Yogurt salad dressing or a Greek Yogurt desert.

Another suggestion for adding more variety to a pasta meal is to add any of a variety of vegetables to the pasta for a change in flavor as well is making a dish that is more colorful and festive.

➢ **BOILED EGGS** made ahead, provide a number of ideas for quick light meals.

➢ **BOILING A POT OF POTATOES** and keeping them in the refrigerator is a great way to add extra variety to a quick meal.

➢ **CHEF'S SALAD** A chef's salad can be very filling and quickly made using prewashed salad greens, boiled eggs, tomatoes, onions and any other vegetable you wish to add such as zucchini, eggplant croutons etc.

➢ **SAUCY BROWN RICE** "Microwave in the bag brown rice" topped with "microwave in the bag vegetables" and picante sauce; served with hummus, boiled eggs and a side salad of prewashed salad greens makes a delicious saucy meal.

➢ **HOT POTATO SURPRISE** Besides being a good side dish, a baked potato can also be made a quick lunch by slicing it in half and using a fork to chop up the inside of the potato.

To this you can add various toppings of your choice such as: cottage cheese, shredded cheese, chopped nuts, onions, and variety of seasonings such as onion powder, basil or parsley.

Adding prewashed salad greens for a side salad makes for a great lunch.

➢ **VEGGIE TORTILLA** Flour tortillas or corn tortillas make for a very festive meal. Heat the tortilla by placing it on a hot ungreased pan and heat until lightly browned. Remove from heat and rollup rather tightly for a minute.

You can now add prewashed salad greens, shredded cheese, black beans (well-drained), diced onions, sweet peppers or any veggies you have on hand.

Add some picante sauce and top with some sour cream or sweetened plain Greek Yogurt. Now roll them up for a great quick tasty meal.

> **PITA BREAD SANDWICH** To pita bread, add a handful of leaf lettuces and use your imagination for a great sandwich.

You can add Tomato, onion, shredded cheese, boiled eggs, any veggies of your choice and top with a sauce and sour cream or sweetened plain Greek Yogurt... Enjoy!

> **CREAMY SWEET POTATO** Sweet potatoes are a great alkaline food.
Rinse the sweet potatoes well and wrap in parchment paper to bake in a microwave or in aluminum/parchment paper and bake in a conventional oven.

While still hot, cut the sweet potato in half lengthwise. Now add either cottage cheese, sweetened plain Greek yogurt, sour cream or cream cheese.
Complement this with a side salad for a tasty light meal.

> **SWEET POTATO/BROCCOLI BAKE** To a baking sheet lined with aluminum foil and sprayed with nonstick oil:
Add Sweet potatoes (chopped into large chunks... with skin left on) plus lots of broccoli (frozen or fresh) in amongst the chunks of sweet potatoes.

Sprinkle lots of sliced onion (separated into ringlets) over the sweet potatoes and broccoli.

Cover lightly with aluminum foil. Bake at 450° (about one hour) or until potatoes are just getting somewhat tender.

Remove foil and bake another ten or fifteen minutes...just

long enough to lightly brown the vegetables (watch them carefully these last few minutes; so they do not burn).

You can add sour cream, cream cheese hummus or even picante sauce...whatever you are in a mood for. Make lots of this/it goes very quickly (Even people who don't like sweet potatoes actually love this).

➤ **FRUITY GREEK YOGURT** Plain Greek yogurt, a great protein source, can be a tasty, nutritious, quick breakfast by adding Stevia, and fresh or frozen fruit of your choice.
For some extra fiber you can add some pecans or walnuts.

➤ **CREAMY SAUCE TOPPING** Use plain Greek yogurt mixed with either hummus or a very small amount of mustard. If you wish, you can add spices to taste (onion powder, garlic powder, basil, cilantro, parsley etc.). Add Stevia to taste and blend well. For a great, high protein sauce, spoon over rice, baked potatoes, cooked broccoli etc.

➤ **HIGH PROTEIN CREAMY SALAD DRESSING** It can be as simple as just blending a few packets of stevia and a couple tablespoons of water into plain Greek Yogurt and using it to top a veggie salad or as an excellent dip for fruit chunks.
For a more complex version, you can add a few of your favorite herbs and spices before using it to top your veggie salad. This thick high-protein dressing is so simple to use and so versatile.

After you have worked out a menu of foods that are easy for you to prepare, make a list of the ingredients used in the ones that you will use most frequently. Keep this list on hand so it will be easier to prepare a shopping list when a flare up does occur.

CHAPTER 10
REDUCING STRESS

"How do you avoid stress when it follows you throughout your life?"

You hear repeatedly that individuals with fibromyalgia must avoid stress because it can result in an increase in fibromyalgia symptoms and possibly flare-ups.

We hear this and yet we wonder, "How are we going to avoid the unavoidable?" Things happen. Besides the stress of pain, that we live with each day, life and its surprises must be contented with.

People we love become ill, unexpected bills arrive at least convenient times, houses develop expensive repair problems, some people in our lives are difficult to get along with, bosses make illogical demands, we get laid off, or worse than that, we lose jobs.

"So how is it possible to avoid stress?"

Although there is no way of removing stressful situations from your life, there are basically three ways of coping with this stress, and they must be used together. These are "stress reduction", "stress avoidance" and stress-relieving supplements.

STRESS REDUCTION

I wish there were easy answers for all the problems in your life, but for the ones that are not easy to deal with, the one thing you can do is try to keep them from affecting your health. The better you feel, the easier it is to deal with life's ups and downs.

"Take a break." "Do what you can do for now." If there is nothing else you can do for now, dwelling on the problem will not make it go away; it will only make you feel worse (physically and emotionally).

Getting your mind absorbed in something else so it can relax will help for a while. This may give your mind the break it needs in order to see the problem more clearly and handle it much better.

This in no way means that you give up on the problem at hand, just give your mind the chance to relax when the problem seems overwhelming; then you will be able to accept the situation and find a way to cope with things that cannot be changed.

HOW TO RELAX YOUR MIND

Your mind needs time to relax even if for only a short time, in order to deal with stress. Now how do you rest your mind?

Your mind likes to think. If you are at rest, what is your mind usually "doing"? It is usually doing busy work like figuring out a grocery list, deciding what to make for dinner etc.

But one thing the mind seems to come back to repeatedly is the rehashing of problems. It just does not want to let things go until a solution has been reached.

You will need something for your mind to think about in order to get it off whatever is causing you to feel stressed.

Have you ever had a pain that had been bothering you but you just sort of put it in the back of your mind as you talked with some friends. Then suddenly, someone thoughtfully asked how you were feeling and instantly the pain was back and you retorted, "Thanks for reminding me". Your mind had been absorbed in conversation with your friends; it was overlooking your immediate pain until you were reminded of it again.

The same principle applies to things that cause us mental stress. You need to give your mind a break "an escape...something to think about".

Your escape should be something that is "thought absorbing" like taking a brisk walk, watching a sitcom, tossing a ball for your dog, taking a relaxing bath, doing some kind of mind challenging puzzle, playing a game, reading a good book, writing, painting etc.

Now your mind is doing what it likes to do best...thinking. But you have given it something that *you want it to think about*, something it can become thoroughly absorbed in if you let it. You have to learn to completely let go; train yourself to let your mind become absorbed, even if for only a brief time, in what you are doing instead of bouncing back to the problem that is causing your stress.

If your mind is given the break it needs to heal, you may see the problem more clearly and handle it much better.

HOW TO LET GO OF STRESS

Besides the idea of giving your mind the rest it needs for those unavoidable stressful events in life, there is also another complication that we often seem to overlook. This is the stress brought on by our own attitudes.

Your own thought patterns can have a very powerful influence on your attitude. Changing the direction of these thought patterns from negative to positive may not change your situation, but it will give you a better attitude toward things that would normally have stressed you out.

For example: if you are troubled by something that, in the future, "might" affect you negatively and there's absolutely nothing you can do right now to change it, then you create in your mind the most positive outcome for that matter that you can imagine, and then let it go. You are not hiding your head in the sand and refusing to face reality. The problem is not even "real" yet. It is only, at best, a "maybe".

Everyone has problems to deal with and we cannot ignore them. We have to ask ourselves "is there anything that I can do today to help correct this?" If there is something you can do, then do it now. If there is nothing you can do, dwelling on that problem will not make it go away. Get your mind absorbed in something else.

Have you ever heard people say something like "When I am nervous, I have to bake something," or "I have to clean house, or I have to clean closets". These are healthy outlets for stress. These people are doing something to get their minds onto something else for a while; they are giving themselves some healing time.

Everyone has something they benefit from doing during times of stress; it can be a hobby or any other avenue of keeping busy.

The cause of stress is still there, but it is much easier to deal with when using these healing times of stepping outside of the issue that is causing the stress.

TAKING A MENTAL BREAK

Besides the stress of daily life, there is of course, the stress brought on by the fatigue and pain signals bombarding your body day and night. It is only normal to feel slightly overwhelmed at times.

During times of increased pain, you have probably noticed that the more symptoms you are experiencing, the easier it is to become agitated and stressed out...especially over little things.

Stress is what we make of it. How we handle it is very important. Too often we let things stress us out and end up with a flare-up and wonder "why?" We have to practice "letting go" of stress.

AVOIDING STRESS USING A NEW POINT OF VIEW

There is no certain way to handle stress; you have to find out what works best for you. You are responsible for your reactions to people and situations.

Dr. James Dobson once said, "There are very few certainties that touch us all in this mortal experience, but one of the absolutes is that we will experience hardship and stress at some point." Stress may be inevitable, but how we handle it is our choice.

Some people find time spent with their family to be stressful. There are some people that we love that are more prone to bother us than others are.

However, we need the strength and the support of family and friends more now than ever before. There is no greater gift that they could give than to be there when we need them.

We love our families, but like us, our families are not perfect. So try to see areas that cause the most stress for you and work on plans for making the times with your family less stressful. This may mean swallowing your pride and not saying what is on your mind. Just because you are right about something does not mean you are right in saying it. And you know what? After all is said and done you will likely be glad that you kept your mouth shut.

If you are fortunate enough to have friends and family living nearby, let them know that they are welcome, but ask if they could call ahead just in case you're having a bad day.

If having company truly proves to be too stressful for you, then perhaps, you would feel less stress by visiting them, instead, so you can go home when you're tired.

SMILING CAN BE THERAPEUTIC

Do more things that make you smile. These could be things like playing with a pet, watching a comedy on TV or movies that make you laugh; especially if you can share the laugh with others.

Try sharing a smile with another person and see how that makes you feel good inside. Smiling can be very therapeutic. It gives you a release from tension and helps you to feel released from stress.

Medical News Today reported on the latest study conducted by Kraft and Pressman. In the study, they invited 169 volunteers from a Midwestern university to undergo an experiment in two stages: training and testing.

Using various stress inciting activities, they instructed the groups to each perform the activities while holding various facial expressions.

The groups that were instructed to hold slight smiles, forced smiles and all out big happy smiles involving the use of eye muscles, all came out well ahead of the groups that had somber expressions Etc. They had a lower heart rate and were less stressed out than the other groups.

Stress definitely does affect our health by decreasing the serotonin activity in our brain; thus throwing our whole body chemistry out of whack.

There are many stress relieving techniques and supplements that do help. You could talk to your naturopathic doctor or nutritionist about finding help (not sales persons). Tell them about your concerns and they can guide you to what is right for you.

"Remember that stress
doesn't come from
what's going on in your life
it comes from
your thoughts about
what's going on in your life."

Andrew Bernstein

CHAPTER 11
COPING WITH MEMORY PROBLEMS

Memory problems are a very real and very frustrating part of fibromyalgia. These memory problems can even become so pronounced as to make some people fear they have Alzheimer's.

What we need to understand is that unlike Alzheimer's disease, the memories are still there, just slow in coming to the surface.

The brain is easily "muddled" by the condition of the body. Anything from allergies to insomnia can affect the delicate networking and intra-communication abilities of the brain.

You could compare the human brain to the workings of a computer. You know how everyone has days when his or her computer is slow. All it takes, sometimes, is for the computer to run a virus check in the background, for everything to run super slowly.

Many things can possibly account for this human "brain drain" such as:

- The stress from pain and fatigue
- Related illnesses, like thyroid disorders etc.
- Lack of restorative sleep
- Depression
- Various medications, even Benadryl

There are various ways that these problems with the brain can manifest themselves as a sort of "mental fatigue":

- As fibro fog that is known to appear at a certain time of day; especially when fatigue and other symptoms are usually at their worst.

- Short term memory loss

- Fuzzy thinking (sort of like when you have a bad head cold and you're not thinking that well).

- Disorientation that causes familiar surroundings to seem unfamiliar.

- Mental confusion that makes it hard to grasp ideas

- Difficulty concentrating

- Hard to concentrate

- Difficulty learning new things

This mental fatigue, referred to as "fibro fog" or "fuzzy thinking", can be very disabling. Causing you to do a lot of "just standing around and not knowing why you are there and what you should do next". Fibro fog can be very upsetting to the person experiencing it, especially if they do not know what it is.

The extent of the fibro fog you are experiencing is usually in proportion to the extent of pain, stress or fatigue that you are also experiencing. Depending on the severity of the fibro fog you are experiencing, you can suffer from any or all the symptoms of mental fatigue mentioned above during your worst hours of the day.

Though you may experience various degrees of fibro fog at different times, it is usually worse at one certain time of the day.

Fibro fog is especially noticeable when you are very tired, having more pain than usual or during flare-ups.

Some people have it worse for an hour or so after they awaken in the mornings, and some people have it worse in the evenings after a long tiring day. Some people have it both ways but it is usually worse at the same time(s) each day.

Since fibro fog does seem to be predictable, to an extent; you can, sometimes, prepare for it by saving jobs that require mental clarity for the time of day when your mind is at its best.

Another way to lessen the problems caused by fibro fog is to be prepared for it by writing out a very detailed list of activities usually performed at this particular time of day when fibro fog seems to be at its worst.

For instance, if the brain fog is worse in the morning when you are doing your morning routine; make a detailed list of your regular morning habits.

Do not write "put on the teakettle and get breakfast foods out of refrigerator". Write this list out giving very detailed instructions one step at a time rather than combining steps.

At a time of day when you are at your best, look this list over and add extra steps where you see the need for them. After a few days of repeating this procedure, you should have your list the way you want it.

Do not leave any small detail out or you will end up not turning on the teakettle, leaving bread in the toaster oven not toasted, or even worse yet, a stovetop not turned off.

EXAMPLE OF BEGINNING A FIBRO FOG LIST:

1. Pour cold water into teakettle
2. Put teakettle onto the stovetop's right front burner
3. Turn on the right front burner to medium heat
4. Go to refrigerator
5. Get "four" items from the refrigerator: bread, butter, eggs and jam (it helps your memory to count things).
6. Get out the small skillet

Without the list, you may find yourself doing something like just standing in front of the open refrigerator door for a long period of time with your mind on some completely unrelated subject (or on absolutely nothing at all). Then when you "come to" you have no idea why you are standing there.

This list keeps you moving along just as you would on a normal day. No one would ever know you had a problem.

Play it safe, make two lists just in case one should get lost. You could also put clear adhesive plastic over them to keep them from becoming dog-eared or stained.

If you are having a problem with severe fibro fog, take heart; this is only for a season of time. The more you learn about handling these severe problems and what may be triggering them, the less severe they usually become and the less often you will have these episodes.

MY PERSONAL EXPERIENCE WITH FIBRO FOG

When I first started experiencing severe fibro-fog, it was out of necessity that I came up with the idea of making a list. Without the list, I was absolutely "lost".

I literally did not know what to do next in my morning routine of preparing breakfast, and my mind would wander so unremittingly that it would take forever to do a simple 15 minute morning routine. Even then, I would usually forget to do something. I hung onto this list like my life depended on it.

I made the list out during a time of day when I had a clearer head. The next morning I followed the list and then, later in the day, I jotted down anything that I needed to go more into detail on. After a few days, I had a great task list to follow. I then covered it with clear adhesive plastic.

By the time I finally no longer needed the list, I had gone through two of these lists and the second list was already becoming wrinkled and dog-eared.

During this time that I had these severe memory problems, a psychologist misdiagnosed me as being in the early stages of Alzheimer's.

This was many years, and what seems like a lifetime, ago. As I learned to "adjust" my life around the peculiarities of fibromyalgia, the memory problems became less and less.

One reassuring note I can add is that one doctor told me not to be concerned; "persons with Alzheimer's do not know that they have a memory problem". Their mind is clear, "not foggy". The only good memories that they have are from their childhood or very early adulthood and maybe two or three minutes ago.

EXPERIENCING FIBRO- FOG? SAFETY FIRST

When you are going through a time of memory concerns associated with fibromyalgia, you should "never trust your memory when it comes to safety".

One of the main safety concerns usually involves the kitchen area because of the stovetop. When you go into the kitchen, you need to develop some type of safety procedure to prevent walking out of the kitchen with a stovetop burner left turned on. It does not matter if you are only *"going to leave for a minute"* to toss the clothes into the dryer or to go to the bathroom. If there is something cooking on the stovetop; "turn it off". Better to forget to turn it back on then to forget something is cooking.

- One suggestion for handling this problem is to have a small timer worn about the neck, in your pocket or pinned to your shirt. Upon entering the kitchen, you can set the timer button to go off in 10 or 15 minutes, but do not click the "start button" until you have to leave the kitchen "for just a minute".

There are many very good clock/timers suitable for wearing about the neck etc. "Polder" is just one example of a company that manufactures such timers.

(For safety, you may wish to purchase a neck strap that has a breakaway or magnetic clasp in place of the one that comes with the timer. These can usually be found in the sporting goods section of most local department stores.)

"NEVER TRUST YOUR MEMORY WHEN IT COMES TO FIRE SAFETY."

Using a timer may sound unnecessary and overly cautious. But if you accidentally get involved in something else, you may not think of the stovetop until two hours later when you notice your home is engulfed in smoke and flames.

Do not underestimate the damage that the subtle "<u>Oh, I will remember this</u>" or "<u>Oh, I will be right back</u>" can do.

A PERSONAL CLOSE ENCOUNTER

one chilly autumn morning I turned the teakettle on for some hot water. While waiting for the water to get hot, I took a quick bathroom break.

Then I noticed I had not made the bed yet. I made the bed and sat down to take a break and do some reading; the teakettle was now long forgotten.

After a long while, my cat began scratching violently on the bedroom door, wanting in. I opened the door, and was met by my cat, Snuggles, and a deep, thick, black cloud of smoke. The house was so engulfed with smoke that all I could see was a dim spooky orange light in the direction of the kitchen.

The dim orange light turned out to be flames engulfing the teakettle and attacking the wall and the exhaust fan above the stovetop. Luckily, I always kept a small bottle of powdered fire extinguisher right beside the stovetop. Otherwise, in this deep black darkness, I could never have found it.

I turned off the burner and put the fire out (all this, while trying not to breathe). I felt my way to where I knew the door was and, leaving the door open, I ran out onto the sundeck gasping for air.

The sun was shining very brightly outside. There were two very large windows in the kitchen area, but the smoke was so dense that everything had been solid blackness inside the house except for where the flames were.

About 20 minutes later I held my breath as I quickly went back into the house to turn on the exhaust fan above the stovetop and then returned to the sunporch.

When I went into the house, about 20 minutes later, I could now just barely make out a faint glow of dark orange in the direction of where the windows were located. It took two trips, holding my breath, to get the windows all opened up.

Later on I learned that when a house is completely black like this, you only have seconds before the smoke ignites and the house goes up in flames.

I would have died that day if it had not been for my little "short tailed cat, Snuggles". She, incidentally, was fine and lived to the good age of 16 ½ years old (a very loved cat).

So please understand, when you are suffering from fibro-fog or any other memory problems, you must not take any chances. Anything at all that you are doing that could have bad results if you walked away and did not return must be safeguarded.

As I mentioned earlier, one defense against this kind of problem is a timer that you can carry with you either around the neck, in a pocket or pinned to your clothing; there are also some great android apps that make good timers.

You could also get into the habit of doing something easily noticed for a backup; like pulling a chair across the doorway when you go into the kitchen. Then upon exiting the kitchen area, only remove the chair after you have made a stovetop safety check and/or have set your timer.

"Another great help is to make sure that if you use a teakettle, that it is a whistling teakettle with a "very loud whistle".

As an additional note on using timers, if you are having trouble cooking more than one food at a time without burning at least one, try getting a couple of small kitchen timers and setting each one in a safe vicinity of each food being cooked. Set each timer for the amount of time you think each food could go before being checked on while cooking.

MORE MEMORY COPING AIDS

I have read that if you want to remember to do something, to use visualization. With people who have fibromyalgia, the problem is "remembering" to visualize.

It seems that with fibromyalgia, short-term memory problems are more a result of distraction. Because of the many problems going on in the body, such as pain, muscle weakness, exhaustion, depression, brain fog etc., the mind is sometimes just too distracted to use something like visualization.

Now if it works for you, then by all means, use it to visualize a giant red dodo bird standing in your kitchen doorway that won't let you through until you have done all your safety checks.

Another memory aid is to verbalize your intent. If you are at the stove and you need something from the refrigerator, audibly say what it is that you need, before you even turn to get it from the refrigerator.

This saying the name of the item you need or what you intend to do "out loud" helps to reinforce your memory on the short-term. As mentioned earlier, on some occasions it helps to count items or tasks such as:

- "I need three things from the refrigerator." Name them out loud and then go get them.

- "There should be four things in Johnny's lunch bag."

- "I need to take three things with me to the doctor's office."

SIX IMPORTANT MEMORY TOOLS

On the next few pages, you will find a listing of six of the most important memory tools that will help keep your life in focus in spite of reoccurring memory problems.

- **The Daily Reminder List (on refrigerator)**
- **The Personal Telephone Book**
- **The Internet Address Book**

- **The Stress Saver Notebook**
- **The One Year Calendar Planner Book**
- **The Location Reminder (for in the car)**

1. DAILY REMINDER LIST

An excellent memory coping aid is the "Daily Reminder List".

This list is to be used as a reminder to do those little things that make life go more smoothly if not forgotten. This is to avoid the "Oh my, the day is over and I forgot to…" kind of day.

The Daily Reminder List is not a "chore list". This list is for such things as:

- Mail letter
- Call the electric company
- Call Susie about the play
- Order Tommy's book
- Wash Mary's jacket
- Change the oven's light bulb
- Start dinner early
- Play practice tonight
- Record TV special 8:00 PM; channel 8.

These are the kind of things that just make life run a little more smoothly when you remember to do them. These are also the kind of little things that make life stressful if they are forgotten. Resist the urge to add chores to it, or you will undoubtedly neglect checking it.

Put this list where you are most apt to "actually look at it" during the day. The daily reminder list can be kept on a magnetic shopping list tablet on the refrigerator or wherever is best for you. You will have something on this list every day, so where you put it is where you will always know to look.

Four of the essential backup memory aids can be kept in a small basket on your desk where you make out the monthly bills. They are a <u>Personal Phone Book,</u> a <u>Stress saver Notebook</u>, a <u>Calendar Planner Book</u> and a <u>small book for Internet info and Addresses</u>.

The best place for these books is most likely where you make out the monthly bills and as an added help, you could keep some type of small notebook with attached pen in one or two other spots in your home.

There are many digital devices that are great for the uses I describe below, but if I named them they would be outdated within a very short time. For that reason, we will discuss the plain hardcopy type of memory tools here. Besides, it is good to have a hard copy for backup.

Do you have trouble remembering "Who, What, When, Where, How"? Who was I supposed to ask for? Did I pay that bill? What was the name of the book Angie recommended? Where did I put that phone number? What was that password?

2. THE PERSONAL PHONE BOOK

The "phone book" should be a handy size that you feel most comfortable with and large enough to easily be seen. *Though you may use a digital device for your phone numbers and addresses, it is always good to have a hard copy backup.*

To make your phone book (whether digital or otherwise) user-friendly, it is very important that you record the information in such a way that you can find what you're looking for even on those days when you are suffering from fibro- fog.

Instead of racking your brain for the name of a doctor or the last name of an acquaintance, you will enter the listings under the headings that are easiest for you to remember.

Which of the following listings would be easiest for you to look under? Why not just use them all so when you are having one of "those kinds of days" you are covered.

- D... Dr. Miller (Veterinarian)
  V... Veterinarian (Dr. Miller)
  P... Pets (Dr. Miller)

M... Miller, Dr. (Veterinarian)

- S... Smith, Dr.(Rheumatologist)
  D... Doctor Smith, Rheumatologist
  R... Rheumatologist, Dr. Smith

- C... Carter's auto Repair
  A... Auto (Carter's repair)

- J... Johnson, Mary
  M... Mary Johnson
  G...Garden Club, Mary Johnson

- M... Metropolitan Bank
  B... Bank (Metropolitan)

- M... Marietta Hospital
  H... Hospital (Marietta)

Listing new entries properly, at first, and then in the way that is easiest for you to recall them makes a phone book much easier to use on those days when you can't even remember your best friend's last name.

You can also list things of a kind under a group heading such as:

Bank...Metro
Bank...City
Bank...First National

Auto...Bill's repair
Auto...Gary's sales
Auto...AAA

Now your phone book is more user-friendly and you will have fewer times of having to go through your entire phone book for a listing because you are having a problem recalling a person's last name or the name of the veterinarian.

Another very helpful addition to your personal phone book is a notes section. In your physical phone book you can use the address section for such things as the name of the contact at a place of business such as the secretary's name and/or any other information that, out of courtesy, you should be aware of.

In your digital phone book, you can list the same contact's names, and other important information under the "notes" section.

You can also use these sections for jotting down the names of spouses and children of friends and acquaintances; you never know when you're going to have one of those awkward moments when you draw a blank when trying to remember the name of a friend's husband or child.

3. THE LITTLE INTERNET ADDRESS BOOK

A small, sturdy hardback book will work for keeping information such as Internet site addresses, passcodes, usernames, the names of the companies that you bought products from plus serial codes etc. accompanying these products. You will pat yourself on the back for having this as a hard copy backup should something happen to your digital copy or your computer is down (been there, done that). Using small alphabetized tabs, you can organize this little book in the same way as you did with your telephone book…easiest way to recall.

4. THE "STRESS-SAVER NOTEBOOK"

this is definitely a stress saver. It is a handy-sized notebook for jotting down information from phone conversations.

You can jot down little bits and pieces from personal and business calls such as upcoming events, dates, names, etc. that you may need to recall in the future.

You will be amazed at how much stress this little "secretary" will save you. Keep this notebook in the area where you would need it for the majority of your transactions throughout the day.

To Prepare Your Notebook for Use:
- You will draw a two-inch margin line (from top to bottom)-------------- on the outer right side edge on the first page of the notebook. Repeat this process of making an outside margin on the remaining pages of the book.

- You will use this right margin of each page to write down the subject of the phone conversation or name of the person it was with etc.

- Use the left side of the page for jotting down the notes from the conversation.

  You do not have to make "good" notes, just enough to get the gist of what was said in the conversation.

- Make sure to include any names, dates, places, times etc. You can mark where your latest entries are with a paperclip or rubber band. This little book can make you look like a person with a great memory.

  This is especially great when you are ordering something like a service. If your first bill comes and it is for more than you agreed to pay, you now have all the info and the name of the person you spoke to, right there in your stress saver notebook.

  When you call and get everything straightened out by using the information you have in your notes, you can take new notes on this latest conversation; including the name of the person with whom you talked to last. Now if the bill is wrong again, you are ready.

If you do not want to be bothered with making these outside margins in your book, you can use a "planner/organizer notebook" that already has a "project notes" margin on each page.

By turning the planner book upside down and starting from the back, you will have your right hand margin already made for you. These notebooks can be found in various sizes at most office supply stores.

5. A ONE YEAR CALENDAR PLANNER

you can find these planners in many sizes and thicknesses. Find the size that fits into your workspace must comfortably. Here again, you may find it more convenient to go digital; but the idea is the same.

Planners can be used to keep track of bill payments, appointments etc.

If there is a "to do" list in the margin, this is an added plus. It can be used for making notes of annual recurring events such as birthday reminders, insurance premium payments, annual blood tests, annual events etc. At the end of each year, these can be recorded into the New year's calendar book.

On the calendar part, you can mark on the date things like: the confirmation number accompanying payments made, amount paid, doctor appointments etc.

This prevents the scary scenario that often happens three weeks after bill was due. The "did I pay the such and such bill?" It is such a relief to open the planner and see that it was paid and if it was paid by phone, that it has a confirmation number next to it.

6. A LOCATION REMINDER FOR TRAVELING

The last of the six memory aids is "A Location Reminder". This is great for in the car; it avoids the frustration of embarking on a trip to a destination and realizing you have forgotten where it is.

This may be a destination that you travel often, but today you just cannot get a handle on its location no matter how much you search your mind.

Keep a small notebook in your car with a listing of general directions to destinations such as doctors' offices, organizations, malls, people's homes etc.

If this list becomes too large, you may find it more convenient to use a small notebook that has alphabetical tabs.

Next to the name of the destination, add the major road(s) that will take you in that direction. You can add a an exit number, or any other information that you may need in order to find this place. If you feel a map is needed, write "see map".

In the back of the book you can have a place to draw or write maps with more detailed information. You can use this book for places that you visit frequently as well as places you visit only occasionally.

Your Entries Could Read Something Like:

- Town Mall... Route 20, Greenwood exit
- Pediatrician... I- 40, Union Street exit- Camp Road
- Lakewood Center... 50 E. Turn left at Burger King
- Mary Johnson... Hallmark Road*see map
- Hospital... Route 115, Lakewood exit
- Orthodontist... turn right after Lakewood Mall, Old Locke Road
- Johnson's bookstore... next to the Dairy Queen, route 50

Make the location reminder book in a way that is easy for your own personal use. You will probably seldom have to use it, but when you do, you will appreciate the time that you took to make it.

STICKY NOTES

sticky notes are great reminders, but you have to be careful how you use them. A sticky note can sit right beside you on your desk day after day and never be paid attention to. Sometimes you get so used to seeing sticky notes that you actually forget to "look" at them.

One spring day I had the bright idea of using sticky notes to list the outside chores that we had to take care of.

After posting these notes in the shed where I was sure they would be easily seen and handy for accomplishing these tasks, I never thought of them again.

I never noticed these notes until the next spring when I again thought it would be a good idea to use sticky notes and put them in the shed; there they were, the forgotten notes from the year before.

The only way I have found that I can use sticky notes for projects and trust myself to look at them is to put them in a place that I would see them at the start of my day. They can be placed on a TV screen, microwave door, computer monitor etc.

I keep my "daily reminder list" on the refrigerator because I have gotten into the habit of checking here every day. However, if there is something that I have to remember to do right away in the morning, it is a good idea to use the sticky note way.

CALENDAR REMINDERS

for a visual reminder, a good old-fashioned calendar that has ample room to write notes in the squares around each date is handy for birthdays, appointments etc. You can even keep a shallow "notes container" close to the calendar to use for dropping appointment cards into when you return home from a doctor's appointment, vet appointment etc. Transferring the information from the card to the calendar can be one of your "things to do while sitting down" projects.

You can use sticky notes on the calendar for upcoming events scheduled past the new year; then when you replace the old calendar the notes are easily transferred to the new calendar.

You may forget to check the calendar, forget to send the card or keep the appointment until it is too late, but at least the info is there to use; Good Luck!

ALL- IN ONE BOOK

You may find it helpful to keep an "All- In One Book" in which you can record everything from "How to turn on the air compressor", to "How to prepare meals for special occasions". This can also be done on your computer in a "How To Do It" file.

You can keep notes on anything you feel necessary to remember how to do, especially if you would be at a loss without this information. You can even keep such information as a complete shopping list for special occasions and holidays (such as dishes that are more or less a tradition).

It may even be beneficial to keep a list of foods or recipes that family members and friends dislike or like (or maybe have allergies to).

When you keep "How To" instructions; write them as if you were instructing someone else on how to do this. If you have to refer to your notes, "you probably have forgotten how to do them".

You can label each file or section of your book with categories such as "How To", "Holidays", "Recipes", "Computer tips" etc.

ELECTRONIC MEMORY AIDS
In this computerized age, there are many portable digital devices out there that you can use as memory aids; you just have to find the one that best suits your needs.

There are also programs and apps that you can use on your computer. These programs offer numerous memory aids for just about everything I discuss in the section about memory.

Some of these programs are perfect for recording information related to flare-ups.

NEUROBIC EXERCISES FOR THE MIND
Neurobics is a rather new concept. It is the science of exercising the mind to keep it fit and to prevent its deterioration. These exercises have nothing in common with the puzzles and brainteasers that one normally associates with brain exercises; although these puzzles do offer important challenging exercises for the brain.

Neurobics deals with the part of the brain that:
- Learns new things
- Accesses stored memories
- Makes associated linkings

Neurobics deals with problems such as memory lapses, forgetfulness and mental confusion; problems normally related to persons with fibromyalgia and aging seniors.

University of Michigan psychologist Denise Park, a specialist in the field of cognition in the aging, reported on a new study of cognitive functioning in fibromyalgia patients that was funded by the Arthritis Foundation and the NIH National Institute of Arthritis and

Musculoskeletal and Skin Diseases (NIAMS).

Dr. Park and her scientific team discovered that persons with fibromyalgia had cognitive functions similar to adults 20 to 30 years their senior. This was obviously due to the brain's overload of info resulting from constant pain, excessive fatigue, and other factors known to interfere with concentration and memory.

In the book "Keep Your Brain Alive", by L. C. Katz.PhD & M. Rubin, you will find some interesting examples of neurobic exercises.

Neurobics involves the use of the five senses and emotion. The exercises are geared toward alternately changing the way you carry out daily routines; doing them in ways unlike those ways in which you are accustomed.

You are to find ways to use all of the five senses every day to aid you in your task of building up your network of memories and memory retrieval.

Hopefully some of these memory suggestions will prove helpful to you in your daily struggles with memory problems. I wish you every success.

CHAPTER 12
SUNLIGHT, TRAVEL AND SOCIAL COMMITMENTS

Getting out of your normal surroundings will often give you the lift that you need when you have to endure another day of battling fibromyalgia.

Sunlight travel and social commitments can be very beneficial for people who have fibromyalgia as long as they are careful to not over extend themselves and to always keep their priorities in check.

While it is true that travel and social intervention may be difficult for a person with health problems, they do usually prove to be very uplifting and rewarding in the long run.

In this chapter we will discuss some helpful ideas on these subjects that you may wish to consider.

Living in the North Eastern United States, I can really appreciate the way a bright day of sunshine can make you feel after a long siege of cold winter weather.

Suddenly the sun breaks out; bringing with it a rise in temperature and it seems you can feel the icicles from the winter doldrums melting within you just as assuredly as you can see the icicles and snow melting under the sun's warm rays outside your window.

There is no doubt in my mind that the sun brings healing to our souls as well as to our bodies. You should make an effort to go outside every single day (weather permitting). This will give you the lift that you need when you have to endure another day of battling fibromyalgia.

If there is a problem with sun sensitivity, going outside very early in the morning or at least early in the evening may be your best choice.

If you are bedbound, you could ask someone to pull you over to a window (preferably an open window). If you can sit in a wheelchair, ask someone to assist you in going outside at least once a day (weather permitting).

What is even better than sitting in the sun is to take an invigorating walk in the sunshine. Taking along a buddy to enjoy the sunshine with you always seems to increase your enjoyment; this can be a friend or pet.

Be sure to take proper precautions when walking to protect yourself. You should walk in a safe environment and remember to protect your joints and muscles by using whatever ambulatory aid that is at your disposal.

If you are experiencing pain in your hips and/or legs, give them support by using some sort of aid such as a walker or cane (or even two canes if you have problems with your balance or until your legs seem stronger).

SHARING THE OUTDOORS WITH FAMILY AND FRIENDS

Do not feel that you are homebound or unable to "do things" with your family. If you want to enjoy a day of shopping, many department stores are beginning to supply customers with wheelchairs and electric shopping carts.

If your family is going on an outing, plan how you can go along. Most amusement parks and theme parks have electric carts available to rent by the day. Many larger zoos will have either electric carts or trams that stop at every exhibit center.

Be sure to take along anything that will make the trip more comfortable and less stressful, such as a travel pillow, sunglasses, bottled water etc. Be sure to make a list of the items you will be taking with you, including any medications that you may need. Check this list when you pack to go and again when you pack to return, so you do not forget something that you may need on the return trip.

PREPARING FOR TRAVEL

Allow yourself time to prepare for travel. The more time you allow for being prepared, the less stressful the trip will be.

If this is going to involve extensive travel, then it will require more planning. One thing you should include in your planning is time to rest before you leave, and time to rest when you return.

It always helps to have something with you that can occupy your mind if you have to sit for a long length of time. This comes in handy if there is a layover, or when you feel you need to rest.

If you take along something to entertain yourself with, such as a book or magazine, be sure to consider the size and weight of these items. Things have a way of seeming to quadruple in weight when you have to carry them for a long length of time.

Digital gadgetry can be great, and in some cases, a digital reader might be better than carrying a book around. If you do go digital, keep in mind that if your intent is to play games, some games will require Wi-Fi and this may not be available in all areas.

TRAVEL HINTS

If you are traveling by car, be sure to stop often and do some walking about so you will not be stiff and sore by the time you reach your destination.

If you are traveling by plane and the flight is longer than an hour, there is usually ample room for some simple leg stretching exercises. If you do some simple stretches every half hour or so, it will help alleviate stiffness.

I find that occasionally stretching each leg out under the seat in front of me about four times per leg and then raising each knee about four times each (like marching, but in a sitting position) and then doing the stretching again, will help immensely to prevent stiffness.

If you are flying economy, you may have more limited leg-room than other seats, but you usually still have room for the simple stretches. Talk this over with your travel agent, as there are some seats in economy class that offer more legroom than others, such as the seats across from the emergency door entrance. "Economy plus" will also give you a little more legroom, but it will cost a little more than economy class.

If you decide to travel by air, put your vanity aside and use a cane when you are going to do a lot of walking (or running) from terminal to terminal.

Because I have fibromyalgia plus rheumatoid arthritis in both knees and hips and feet, I usually use two canes during air travel as this helps me to walk on the slick floors of the airline terminal without falling or possibly suffering a fibromyalgia flare up later on.

You may find it best to advise your travel agent of your need for a wheelchair. This will often result in you getting a seat on the flight with more legroom. Then when you check in "online" the day before your flight, you may be given the option of choosing seating that has more leg room. These seats vary in prices, but usually start at about $25 extra per seat.

When you first go into the terminal and check your baggage, most airlines will assist you by getting a wheelchair for you and pushing you to the front of the line in the security check and then will take you to your flight gate so you can be one of the first to board. Make sure to mention to the attendant, before each boarding, that you will need a wheelchair when you reach your destination.

They usually automatically make these arrangements, but this may be overlooked unless you mention it before each boarding. By taking time to mention this before each boarding, you will be met by an attendant with a wheelchair or some other accommodations at your next stop and escorted to your next flight connection.

At one of the nation's largest airports, I had to make connections with another airline on the other side of the airport and on a different level. This very efficient airline had a tram to meet me (I would never have made it to my next flight connection in a wheelchair…it would have been a challenge for even a marathon runner).

It was a very interesting tram ride and you had to hang on tightly to your seat (you could tell that the driver liked his job immensely). Even with "Evel Knievel" at the wheel, I just made it to my destination in time.

Another tip for air travel is to pack as much as you can, even purse contents, into your large suitcases. Then keep only absolute essentials with you in your purse or carry-on baggage: two doses of pain medication, maybe a self-inflating neck pillow, cell phone, money, ID and boarding passes, in a small, lightweight shoulder bag or purse. This keeps your hands-free, lightens your load and is much less confusing and less time-consuming.

If you are going to be staying at a motel or hotel, you should ask what provisions for accessibility they can provide for you, such as a ground-floor room or a room close to an elevator.

If you are going to be walking, especially on uneven turf like in a carnival or fair, take along a cane that you feel comfortable using.

Using a money belt can be a plus as this frees your hands for other things. If you are going to be doing a lot of sight-seeing, you might also consider taking along a type of "three-legged folding stool". You can take these little three-legged stools along with you most anywhere. Some fold up to look about like an umbrella and are very light weight. Most open out into a very convenient stool (18 to 26 inches high) that you can use almost anywhere and on just about any solid surface, sand, grass or ground.

These three-legged stools come in various sizes and weight tolerances. You can find them online, and at sporting goods stores (be very sure the weight tolerance is more than sufficient).

You can go onto the Internet and search for "three-legged fold up stools". Before selecting any certain brand, be sure to check out customer reviews on the Internet; this is the best way to avoid unpleasant surprises.

SOCIAL INTERACTION

Being involved in something outside the home can have a very positive effect on you physically and emotionally.

For one thing, social events get your mind off yourself and the problems surrounding fibromyalgia. It also allows you time to interact with others. Depending on the circumstances, it often seems that being in a different setting will also increase your energy levels somewhat.

Social involvement can be as simple as going to church once a week, meeting a friend for coffee once in a while, or taking a walk down the street and back occasionally (weather permitting) and greeting neighbors as you go.

CHOOSING YOUR PRIORITIES WISELY

Everyone has to choose, at times, those things that are highest on their list of priorities to become involved in. When you have fibromyalgia, you may have fewer choices to choose from, and deciding where your priorities lie is a critical decision.

Nevertheless, this does not rule out any social involvement at all. If you see your health or anything high on your list of priorities suffering, then you may have to cut back on the number of activities or just be involved in the same activities but in a different capacity.

Social involvement, especially if it gets you out of your regular surroundings for even a short time, can help you deal with the problems you face with fibromyalgia by boosting your morale, reducing stress and even helping with memory problems.

If you were asked to do something that you feel would be too much for you to handle, just a simple, "I'd love to help but I'm limited as to how involved I can be because of health reasons" should be sufficient.

If you would really like to help, you may ask if you can just "help out" here and there instead of being obligated to fill in a position at a specific time and place.

If you feel an explanation is necessary, you may explain, "Fibromyalgia often flares up with no warning and I don't want to disappoint anyone who would be depending on me to be there at a certain time or even at all."

You may also add that anything you do cannot involve standing or sitting for long periods of time.

You only have so much energy; use it wisely, and in ways that make your life feel fulfilled.

TALKING ON THE TELEPHONE
There is no rule of what "social involvement" has to be, but it should get you out of your environment if it is going to be of a great benefit to you.

Chatting with friends and relatives on the telephone is not a good example of social involvement because this does not get you out of your surroundings. Actually, it seems that chatting on the telephone can even be a rather stressful activity.

Talking on the telephone can be stressful for people with fibromyalgia for several reasons.

When you talk on the telephone:
- You have to be more conscious of the words you use and how you use them (this can be difficult if you often have problems with finding the "right words").

- When you talk face-to-face, you may not realize it, but you actually use body language, to a large extent, to help convey what you are trying to say. You cannot do this over the telephone.

- Sitting down, talking for a length of time in one place, and holding a telephone to your ear can often leave you feeling stiff and sore afterwards.

- Chatting on the telephone with a friend that you are close to and see often, is not so difficult as talking with someone who lives too far away for you to see them often.

- Talking to someone that you seldom talk to can be a little more stressful because you must pay closer attention to what is being said and you may find it harder to keep the conversation going. This can be difficult if you are having a hard day with fibromyalgia symptoms.

HELPFUL HINTS FOR WHEN TALKING ON THE TELEPHONE:

- Being prepared for a phone conversation can take a lot of pressure off of you; especially if the call is of a more formal type. In this case, it helps a lot if you write out a script of what you want to say ahead of time.

- Break the script up into several paragraphs so it is easier to find the information quickly without getting flustered; write this script in larger and very legible letters.

- If your conversation is with a friend or relation it is more likely to be lengthy. So it may be helpful to use the "speaker phone".

  By using the speaker phone, you can get up and walk around while talking and not cause your neck and body to get stiff from holding the telephone. You can also feel free to talk with your hands. The person you're talking to cannot see you using your hands, but if it helps you to do so; then go for it.

- Personally, I have found it to be very beneficial when talking to a friend, to go outside (on a nice day) for the duration of the phone call.
  If you wish, you can even walk to the mailbox or just go for a walk as you talk. You are getting your time outside and you are sharing it with a friend. Just be careful if you are walking while talking that you are aware of your surroundings in order to avoid an accident.

- I have had friends to call me when they are on a long drive. They just put their cell phone in its holder and put it on speakerphone. This breaks up the boredom of a long interstate drive and helps keep them awake and alert as they drive.

So as you can see, sunlight, travel and social commitments are very beneficial in the lives of those who have fibromyalgia as long as they are careful to not overextend themselves and always keep their priorities in mind.

Just be careful to consider your priorities and do not overextend your capabilities.

Very little is needed

To make a happy life,

It is all within yourself,

In your way of thinking.

Marcus Aurelius

****

What you do today

Can improve all your

Tomorrows

Ralph Marston

****

CHAPTER 13
SETTING GOALS FOR A HEALTHY LIFESTYLE

The alternative to not setting goals is finding yourself, in two years, in exactly the same place that you are now (or worse).

Setting goals is highly recommended for anyone, but it is essential for anyone who has a debilitating illness like fibromyalgia.

When you are caught up in the dilemma of living daily life with all the frustrating symptoms of fibromyalgia, it is very easy to be prone to not do anything that takes you out of your comfort zone.

Nonetheless, when you are dealt a heavy blow like fibromyalgia, it is all too easy to become so overwhelmed that it is hard to imagine ever regaining any semblance of a normal life beyond that little thread of hope that there is a medicine out there that will do it all and "Presto!" You will have your life back to normal again.

Writing your goals down and keeping track of your progress, at least once a month, will help you immensely because it gives you conscious and subconscious inspiration to continue what you have started. This encourages you to continue on in spite of flare-ups and days when you're feeling "down" emotionally.

The alternative to not setting goals is finding yourself, in two years, in exactly the same place that you are now (or worse).

No matter where you are in your symptoms, you can do something toward regaining a more active lifestyle right now. It may be a very slow progression at first, but ask yourself, "Isn't even the smallest gain better than staying the same or getting worse"?

There are beneficial changes that can help you reach your goals. These changes will not cure fibromyalgia, but they can give you more energy, a better outlook, less pain when you move, a better overall feeling and maybe a lot less stress in your life.

Discuss the suggestions listed below with your doctor, who is aware of your health history, and ask what changes would be safe for you to incorporate into your lifestyle.

PACING

Pacing your activities will prove to be the most essential part of your progress in reaching your goals. I never felt so inspired as when I found that by simply using pacing, I could once again do many things that I used to do on a regular basis.

It was a gradual process as I incorporated pacing into every part of my daily routine. With pacing, I was, once again, able to clean house, cook, prepare holiday meals, keep up on the laundry, and enjoy outings with my family. I just had to be careful to follow the pacing guidelines and recognize when my body needed rest and respect my limitations.

EXERCISE

Mild exercise is great because it not only makes you stronger (resulting in less painful overall body movement); it also helps to ward off depression by supplying more serotonin to the brain.

Tell your doctor and nutritionist what it is that you would like to accomplish. There are many therapists that can work with you to figure out a program for you to follow.

SUPPORTING YOUR IMMUNE SYSTEM

Most people with fibromyalgia seem to have a problem with their digestive tract and this causes less absorption of essential vitamins, minerals, fats etc.

This is why it is so important for persons with fibromyalgia to supplement these essentials in their diet by proper eating as well as in supplement form.

Your digestive tract is your first physical line of defense against autoimmune illness, or any illness for that matter. There are several steps to discerning just what your body personally needs in order to restore a healthy digestive tract.

To begin with, in the digestive process, chewing your food well allows the digestive enzymes in your saliva to mix with your foods and liquids. This begins the process of digestion right in your mouth, so do not be in a rush when you eat. Relax and chew your food thoroughly.

GLUTEN-FREE DIET

Many people with autoimmune dysfunctions, such as fibromyalgia, find that they have a sensitivity to gluten in their diets (either as an allergy or as gluten intolerance). This problem manifests itself as diarrhea, cramping, bloating, heartburn etc.

Although one single diet will not do the same for all fibromyalgia patients, it has been proven that various changes in people's diets can definitely make a huge difference in the majority of fibromyalgia sufferers' lives.

AVOIDING INFLAMMATION

If you are having a problem with inflammation, it is important to avoid eating those things that are known to promote inflammation.

Protein from meat sources is known to promote inflammation because animal fat contains a compound that the body uses to create inflammation naturally. The US News reported that diets lower in this molecule have been shown to lower inflammation in rheumatoid arthritis patients.

If you eat plenty of vegetables, whole grains and legumes, it is not difficult to get enough protein without eating any animal foods at all. I am not suggesting that you need to become a strict vegetarian; I just want to point out how easy it is to get all the protein in your diet that you actually need without solely resorting to animal protein.

Most one serving sizes of vegetables and whole-grain pastas average about 6 to 8 grams of protein each; even a medium-sized potato has 5 g of protein.

The amount of protein that your body generally needs should be half what your weight is in pounds. This means that if you weigh 150 pounds, your body needs no more than about 75 g of protein per day.

HYPOGLYCEMIA DIET

Hypoglycemia is another common problem that often accompanies autoimmune dysfunction. If you suffer from blood sugar spikes and lows, eliminating sugar and refined carbs from the diet can show immediate improvements.

Hypoglycemia also leaves you vulnerable to Candida, a yeast infection that thrives on the consumption of sugars and highly refined white flour. If you suffer from Candida or fungal infections, you would definitely do well to remove sugars and highly refined white flour from your diet.

When adding fruits into your diet, use good judgment in choosing fruits that are lowest in fruit sugars. You may find it helpful to keep some kind of a protein snack (low glycemic), like walnuts, to eat in between meals or to accompany a fruit snack.

AVOID USING FOOD ADDITIVES INCLUDING MSG (MONOSODIUM GLUTAMATE) AND NITRATES

These flavor enhancers, found in many processed and frozen foods and in some Asian cuisines, are called Excitotoxins.

They can intensify pain symptoms in many individuals with fibromyalgia. They do this by affecting the NMDA receptors. The same is true of luncheon meats, ham, bacon and other foods containing preservatives such as nitrates.

EATING ORGANIC FOOD

Most people with fibromyalgia have increased chemical sensitivities. Not every food you buy would necessarily have to be organic, but in order to avoid GMO foods, chemicals and polluted soils, there are some foods that should only be used when organic is stated on the package.

RAW FOOD DIET

Raw foods provide fiber and a variety of vitamins and minerals, which are good for just about anyone, including people with fibromyalgia, but there has been no definite study to suggest that raw veggies are better than cooked for people with fibromyalgia. However, one definite advantage is that they do not have additives when eaten raw.

HEALTHY FATS IN THE DIET

Dry skin can be helped by the addition of healthy oils such as coconut oil, olive oil and sea buckthorn oil and can be an aid for many commonly seen problems from hair loss to heart health.

COFFEE, TEA, COLAS

Many fibromyalgia patients turn to stimulants such as caffeine rich beverages including coffee, tea and colas, as a source of energy. However, the boost they get is short-lived and soon turns into fatigue. Caffeine not only raises blood sugar levels; it also soon turns into fatigue and increased cortisol levels.

ADDING MAGNESIUM TO YOUR DIET

Researchers believe that a deficiency in magnesium (found in many green vegetables, beans, and whole grains) can contribute to the muscle pain associated with fibromyalgia. Besides adding magnesium rich foods to the diet, people can take a magnesium supplement to help insure that they are getting the minimal recommended daily value (400 mg for women 500 mg for men). This need for magnesium is often the reason many women crave chocolate; especially around that one time of the month.

In a study by the Nestle Research Center in Switzerland, researchers looked at the effects of eating 1.4 ounces (40 g) of dark chocolate every day for two weeks on blood, urine and measures of stress in 30 healthy adults. Half of the chocolate was eaten midmorning and the other half was eaten midafternoon.

The participant's anxiety levels were determined at the start of the study; blood and urine samples were collected and analyzed at the beginning and end of the two week study.

The results showed that eating dark chocolate daily reduced stress hormone levels in those who had high anxiety levels.

Researchers also say dark chocolate appeared to have beneficial effects on the participant's metabolic and microbial activity in the gut.

ADDING PROBIOTICS

Probiotics and prebiotic's are necessary for controlling many associated conditions such as Candida and fungal infections. Probiotics and prebiotics are absolutely essential if you do any type of exercising; it helps the body handle all the garbage that it has to get rid of as a result of exercising.

KEEP YOURSELF HYDRATED

Keeping your body well hydrated detoxifies your body; helping you to recover from flare-ups. Water can also increase your energy levels and improve mental clarity.

GETTING SUFFICIENT SLEEP

With fibromyalgia, sometimes getting to sleep and staying asleep can be a problem. This problem can often be handled by simply cutting back on daytime naps or turning off the TV and/or computer an hour before bedtime so your body can begin producing the sleepy hormone melatonin.

Sometimes the problem may be as simple as needing a better mattress, or because the room is too hot, too cold or too bright.

You may find taking natural supplements such as magnesium shortly before bedtime may help. Whatever you do, try to find a natural remedy rather than just resorting to prescribed medication that may have serious side effects. There are other natural supplements that are known as sleep aids, but these should only be taken on the advice of a naturopathic doctor or a nutritionist.

REDUCING STRESS

Stress is one of the hardest subjects to approach because it comes in so many forms and what triggers a stressful reaction in one person may not trigger a stressful reaction in another person.

Stress definitely does affect our health by decreasing the serotonin activity in the brain; thus throwing the whole body chemistry out of whack.

There are many stress relieving techniques and supplements that do help. You should talk to your naturopathic doctor or nutritionist (not sales personnel) about finding help. Discuss with them your concerns and they can guide you to what is right for you.

Before taking any kind of supplements for reducing stress, you must be sure the supplements will not conflict with any health problems that you may have or medications that you are taking.

~H O P E~
"When you do nothing,
you feel overwhelmed and
powerless.
But when you get involved,
you feel the sense of
hope and accomplishment
that comes from knowing
you are working to make
things better."
Pauline R. Kezer
…………

~HOPE~
"The very least you can do
in your life is
to figure out
what you hope for.

And the most you
can do is
live inside that hope.

Not admire it from
a distance
but live right in it,
under its roof."

Barbara Kingsolver

CHAPTER 14
SETTING UP A PACING ROUTINE

Respect your limitations, work your daily routines around them and allow yourself the privilege of not being perfect

Pacing is essentially just resting before you have depleted your body's energy levels. I know that sounds like saying "turn right three blocks *before* the traffic light", but by becoming aware of your body's energy levels, it will become easier and easier to recognize your limitations.

If you rest *before* you deplete your body's energy limits, you will "recharge" more quickly and reduce the chances of regrettably increasing the intensity of your symptoms.

Another very important thing you should take into consideration when determining your body's energy limitations, is that contributing circumstances can influence your body immensely. These can include such things as:

- Current state of health
- Increased social interaction
- Holiday festivities
- What you did yesterday
- How well you slept last night
- Your attitude toward what you are doing today
- Any kind of added stress

So do not expect as much out of yourself on days following stressful events or health setbacks. Be patient with your body and give it time to heal when it is being influenced by stressful circumstances.

DEVELOPING A PROPER ATTITUDE

Many of us find it difficult, at first, for pacing to work. The main reason is that we dislike "changing the way we have always done things".

Listed below, are a few of the most common attitudes that can prove to be counterproductive in our daily struggle to get things accomplished:

"Are You a Person Who Likes to Work at a Project Until the Job is Done?"

Although this may sound reasonable; working at a project without pacing yourself will actually work against you. With this kind of reasoning you will find yourself accomplishing less and less because this will cause increased fatigue followed by increased pain.

When you have an illness that affects your energy reserves, you have to learn to live a more disciplined life. By this I mean you have to do more planning rather than just taking the day as it comes. This is easier for some personalities that it is for others; a person who enjoys the freedom of doing things on the "spur of the moment", for instance (like your author), may have a problem with planning most everything ahead of time.

If you will honestly dedicate yourself to protecting your energy reserves, you can still be a "spur of the moment" type of person; especially once you can trust yourself to take breaks during your activities whether you feel like you need them or not.

When you live with daily chronic pain, you find yourself trying to ignore this pain as you go throughout your normal daily activities.

You will now have to start paying more attention to what your body is feeling and how certain activities are more demanding on your body than others.

Taking breaks before you are tired will require shorter breaks (whether you feel you need them or not) and will be less stressful on your body than taking breaks when you are already tired, but you have to learn to pay attention to what your body is experiencing.

There's a common misconception that taking rest periods will cause stiffness and soreness to set in.

Before I began using pacing, I pushed myself to finish whatever I was doing because I knew that once I stopped; I would realize just how stiff and sore I really was.

The half-finished jobs began piling up because of this kind of reasoning.

When you have an illness that affects your muscles and soft tissues, **the two major causes of stiffness and soreness are from not resting often enough or from resting too long at a time**. Rest periods that are over 30 minutes in length will allow stiffness to set in; then you will feel too sore to finish the task.

The new reality is that your body needs these rest periods and by giving your body time to renew itself, you can return to your task with renewed vigor. After a timely rest, you will usually make even clearer decisions on how the job should be done and you will be more apt to see projects to completion than before.

You have to learn to keep a balance; resting before you are tired will require shorter rest periods and will help prevent inflammation.

Some things you get involved in during the day may be more stressful and require more frequent breaks or even longer breaks than another would. In these cases, you may find it helpful to follow the advice stated in the chapter on Stress.

During some of your break periods you may find it helpful to give your mind something pleasant to become absorbed in such as: watching a short sitcom on TV, walking to the mailbox, playing fetch with your dog etc. You are in charge of your break time; enjoy the simple things in life.

Sometimes it is just helpful to spend a few minutes sitting in the fresh air and sunshine (weather permitting). A change of scenery can do a considerable amount of good when you feel any kind of stress.

There are some projects that prove to be just too difficult or stressful to be done at one time. These projects are best broken up into many smaller jobs and spread out over several days or even longer. The one thing you want to keep in mind is to complete each small job. This way you will be more apt to want to pick up where you left off the next time.

In other words, if the project is a really big project and requires making a really big mess, you need to try to go out of your way to break it up into several "orderly messes".

Letting yourself finish each "orderly mess" before starting another will make the whole project less stressful. You will find things will go much easier for you, and you will be much more successful in seeing the project completed.

"I always wanted to stay with the project until it was completed even if it meant staying up late and missing meals to get everything done."

"I changed my way of doing things because, quite frankly, I had to; it was beginning to look like I would never catch up again. I realized how seriously fibromyalgia was gradually changing my life and I was getting "snowed under" as a result."

SETTING UP A PACING ROUTINE

You do not have to let fibromyalgia keep you from living your life and from enjoying the life you live. Just respect your limitations, work your daily routines around them and allow yourself the privilege of not being perfect.

"My husband grew up with a friend who was born with only one normal arm. There are a lot of things that you would say a boy with only one arm could never do: like shooting a bow and arrow, playing football (in high school and in college), shooting a rifle, driving a stick shift car etc. but he did them all and he did them well.

"He recognized his "limitations" and figured out how, by taking these limitations into consideration, he could accomplish his goals one at a time; and he did just that."

It is the same with fibromyalgia. In order to accomplish your goals, you also have to recognize your limitations and work with them and around them. Do not try to ignore them because this usually will just "land you flat on your back" with a flare-up.

APPLYING PACING
This new way of doing your daily work consists of breaking your activities up into timed increments.

Once you start pacing your activities, you will be amazed at the increase in your energy levels. Instead of doing things from start to finish, you'll find it less exhausting and quite productive to break them up into these timed increments.

The length of each increment of time allotted to each session will depend entirely upon what you feel you can physically manage at that time. You are totally in control of this "Pacing" program. It is so flexible that you can change it from day to day or hour to hour if necessary.

The important thing is that now, without worsening your symptoms, you can accomplish those things that are most important to you.

A PACING ROUTINE FOR THE KITCHEN
As author of the "Stop the Yeast Syndrome Cookbook", I can say I love to cook. Cooking healthy meals and creating my own whole-grain breads, cakes and cookie recipes for my family were always very enjoyable experiences for me; especially during the holidays.

But now I would find myself not even halfway through preparing a recipe when suddenly I was in so much pain and so exhausted that I could not go on.

At other times, I would start out feeling fine, as I started making dinner. I would suddenly be so overcome with pain and fatigue that I could not finish making the meal.

The pain was so intense, that leaving the cooking project only half finished, I could barely make my way to my bedroom to collapse onto the bed exhausted and in pain over my entire body.

Cooking Does Not have to be Overwhelming

I eventually came up with the following ways of preparing meals without being totally "wiped out" as a result.

- Make a list of at least three meals that could be made for special family get-togethers that are easily prepared or that can be easily made by spreading the work out over several days or even weeks.

- Make a list of about seven or eight nutritious "regular" meals that can be easily prepared. Break each meal's preparations up into several steps that can be accomplished in intervals throughout the day.

  If some of these or even parts of these meals can be baked in the oven using aluminum foil lined with parchment paper, this can really cut down on cleanup.

- On days when you are really tired or feeling stressed, it always helps to be able to use disposable plates, cups etc. as this lessens your cleanup time.

- You may find that on busy days, such as on weekends, your family may want something special like an occasional pizza or something that is quick to fix.

  Sometimes you may find it necessary to give in to preparing a fast food meal, but be careful that it does not become a habit.

  These kinds of fast foods occasionally find their way into every American home, but overuse of such foods that are high in salt, unhealthy fats, and sugars and highly processed flours are something you must avoid in your diet if you want to avoid an increase in fibromyalgia symptoms.

- If you always enjoyed baking and making meals for large family gatherings, there is a way around this if you look hard for it.

  Check out the chapter on holidays for more help. This, again, is something that you will have to carefully consider. You will have to decide just what it is that you enjoy most about such things and let other people jump in and do what they can to help.

- Vegetables that you use often in your food preparations such as: onions, sweet peppers, celery etc. can be chopped weeks ahead of time and frozen or you can buy them in the grocery store already chopped and frozen.

WHEN I FEEL LIKE BAKING QUICK BREADS OR CAKES, I DO IT IN TWO OR THREE STAGES.

"Since I am gluten intolerant, everything I bake, I bake from scratch. I usually make several batches at a time; so this takes some planning:

1. The first day I combine only the dry ingredients.

If the recipe requires cutting in butter or shortening into the flour, this can be considered your second day's step.

Place the dry ingredients inside a plastic food storage bag and close tightly and refrigerate. You can continue the recipe the next day or wait a couple of days when it is convenient for you to continue.

2. On the second day of preparing the recipe, I will cut in the butter or shortening. When finished, place the ingredients inside a food storage bag and close tightly; refrigerate when finished.

3. On the third day, I combine the liquid ingredients of the recipe. I then add these liquid ingredients to the dry ingredients and "tweak" the recipe a little here and there if needed.

If the dough can be refrigerated, I will refrigerate it and bake it on the fourth day; if not, then it gets baked on the third day.

By following these steps in preparing ahead I was able to, once again, do the baking that I love to do.

Pacing and Social Involvement

When someone lives with constant pain and fatigue, it would be too easy to just retire from any social involvements and just take care of "number one".

If you decide you are in so much pain that you no longer want to do things with friends and family anymore; you will be missing out on the joy of being a part of your loved ones' lives.

You must watch that you are not shutting yourself off from life; it is just too short to give into this kind of thinking.

Find ways to do things with friends and family that you are personally comfortable doing, such as: take along a desert and stop in for tea with a friend, or pick up a movie and a snack and spend a couple of hours watching a movie with friends or family.

If you really try, you will come up with ideas for sharing time with your friends and family that you feel confident will not increase your symptoms.

By making pacing a natural part of your daily life and continuing to practice stress relieving strategies, your life can be more than just limited to your little comfort zone.

Sure, there will be times that you will have to cancel plans, and not keep commitments, but at least you are involved instead of letting life pass you by.

Explain this concept of pacing to your family and friends by telling them "that fibromyalgia affects the muscles and soft tissues in your body so you have to avoid inflammation and stiffness". Tell them how important it is for you to often take brief rests and not sit or stand for too long a period of time.

USING A PACING STRATEGY

What pacing is, essentially, is sandwiching your active periods between inactive periods.

It may take some time to get the hang of how you can effectively incorporate this idea of pacing into your daily life, but it helps immensely once you realize your limitations and do not push yourself beyond them.

Two basic rules of thumb to consider:

1. Maximum time to be active; one hour or as you feel capable

2. Maximum time to be inactive; 30 minutes maximum

Being inactive for over 30 minutes allows pain and stiffness to set in.

So, if "Pain has confined you to your couch", the house is a mess, and you do not see how you could ever get it back to normal again because of unremitting pain and fatigue, there is hope to be had.

One thing you may find helpful is the purchasing of a timer that you can wear on you, in your pocket or around your neck. You can set such timers to go off in timed increments of your choice. By the push of a button (like the snooze alarm on your clock) you can time rest periods as well as active periods throughout the day.

By following the guidelines suggested in the chapters on housecleaning, you will find a way to dig yourself out of your dilemma three minutes at a time or less.

You will be surprised at how much you can accomplish in these very short periods of time. On good days, you may be able to make the "busy time" increments longer than on other days.

I find that when I am having a good day and I feel really well, I tend to spend longer on my feet without realizing it and soon I'm regretting it. For these times, I have found it good to set my timer for 45 minutes to an hour. When timer goes off, I set aside what I'm doing, and take a short (or long) rest before returning to being active again. During inactive times, I can read the newspaper, sit down and pet or play with the cat, clean out a drawer or actually just rest.

It is amazing how just a 2 to 15 minute rest "before" you "feel tired" is often enough to give you the needed strength to continue on for another 45 minutes or so.

TWO IMPORTANT THINGS TO REMEMBER:
- The time for being active can be from one minute to no longer than one hour before taking a rest; even if the rest time is only a short two or three minutes.

- The time for being inactive (sitting down) can be any time between one minute and 30 minutes; but should not exceed 30 minutes in order to avoid a problem with painful stiffness.

You should check with your doctor to see if he agrees that you are physically capable of using pacing and has ruled out any possible illnesses that would prevent you from being active at this time. When you start to use pacing, keep in mind that the less active you have been, the shorter your active times should be.

WAYS TO BE ACTIVE WHILE BEING INACTIVE
Being inactive does not necessarily mean doing nothing at all; you can spend your inactive times doing "busy work while sitting down" such as:

Magazine sorting
Folding clothes
Cleaning out a drawer
Playing with a pet
Watching a movie
Doing crafts
Listening to music
Reading
Drying your hair
Sketching

BEING ACTIVE INCLUDES ANY FORM OF ACTIVITY THAT YOU FEEL UP TO DOING, SUCH AS:
Walking to the mailbox
Playing with a pet
Preparing dinner
Making your breakfast
Tidying up a room
Feeding your pet
Making your bed
Getting a drink of water
Getting dressed

In the chapters on "Housecleaning", you are given tips on how to clean house in small timed increments; the list can be as expansive or as simple as you wish it to be.

Pacing will give you time to do such things as going to church and then sitting down or going to the market and sitting on a scooter to shop. If you go on a trip to the zoo, many zoos have scooters available or trams that travel from site to site; just be sure that you keep a routine of being active and then resting before being active again.

USING NAPS WISELY
Some of your inactive periods can actually be used for a nap when needed. Naps can be an essential part of your healing process, but so is a decent night's sleep. If your naps total more than one hour per day, you will likely find yourself not sleepy at bedtime.

You can break naps up into four naps daily of 15 minutes each or two 30 minute naps or one big one hour nap. Try to make these naps as early in the day as possible. Do not nap close to dinnertime or you are apt to not be sleepy at bedtime.

You should have at least seven hours of sleep at night (preferably eight hours sleep) to increase your chances of going into a restorative sleep phase.

By applying this idea of Pacing into your lifestyle, you will eventually start to feel that you are more in control of your life again.

SCHEDULED REST PERIODS

I have found that taking a scheduled rest period at that time in the afternoon when I begin to tire after lunch, to be very beneficial. I also take a scheduled second rest (not nap) after all the busy work of the evening "rush" is over.

These rest periods do not have to be very long. They can be as short as 15 minutes to as long as 30 minutes; depending on how I feel.

The rest periods are not set aside because I am tired, they are mandatory; even if I am feeling great and do not want to rest, I take these rest periods.

You may not see the reasoning behind this, at first, but in a very short time you will realize what a difference these two rest periods make and how will you feel and how well you sleep at night.

Set your timer so you do not have to keep looking at the clock, close out the world, lie back and rest. This is not for sleep just rest. This is not for TV or reading or anything except complete rest.

Over time, you will begin to look forward to these times that you set aside just for yourself. Eventually, you'll find this discipline carries over into your bedtime regimen and you'll find it easier to relax and fall asleep at your regular bedtime.

Once you put the discipline of practicing this pacing program into your routine, you will be surprised at the difference it makes in your energy levels.

You will find that you can make a big difference if you put out the effort needed and resolve to yourself that the hassle of pacing is worth trying.

CHAPTER 15
CREATING A USER-FRIENDLY ENVIRONMENT

Small changes in our environment can make enormous increases in our activity levels and reduce our fibromyalgia symptoms

Making changes in your life is always difficult, but life-changing illnesses, such as fibromyalgia, eventually do make change necessary as your environment becomes more and more of a challenge for you.

Making your environment user-friendly is possibly one of the most important choices you can make. Besides some major changes in your home, numerous small changes can make impressive differences in both your daily energy levels and pain reduction.

You may find it to your advantage to consult with an occupational therapy practitioner before attempting any changes in your home or workplace.

An Occupational Therapist can come to your home or place of work and help you to decide what changes would be most beneficial for you.

By focusing on the needs of the individual, they can decide not only if you could benefit from various kinds of mobility devices, but also how to adapt your home environment to fit the your individual needs.

By using the therapist's list of recommended changes, you can now decide what changes need to be taken care of immediately and what changes can wait to be done in the future.

Sometimes major home changes are also necessary; you will likely need to seek out a contractor for addressing these major changes.

USE OF MOBILITY DEVICES

There are so many kinds of mobility aids and products made to aid you in your daily living.

Misunderstanding keeps some people from using the very things that have been created for them to be able to live active and productive lifestyles.

Some people refuse to use a cane because they fear it will make their condition worse. This could be true if you were to use a cane improperly.

Talk to your doctor or physical therapist about whether a cane would be helpful or if you should be using a walker of some sort. The most important thing here is how you can keep yourself active with the least amount of danger of falling.

If you normally get around fine without the aid of a cane, then there should be no problem with just using a cane to steady yourself when taking a walk. But leaning heavily on a cane could eventually cause new problems; problems that could be easily avoided by seeking the advice of a therapist.

A cane's main purpose is to help you walk correctly and keep you from falling; as a result, the muscles that help you to walk straight and tall are kept strong in spite of the pain. As these muscles become stronger, you will notice a decrease in the pain as you walk

The same advice goes for all mobility aids; seek the advice of a therapist on how to use the aid properly. If you are not mobile because of pain, you need to seek professional advice on what type of mobility aid would be best for your use.

Although I do not use any aid such as a cane at home, but when walking in the country or uneven sidewalks, I personally use the aid of a cane for the purpose of steadying myself. If I will be walking for a significantly long period of time in crowded areas or over slick floors, (such as in an airport) I will sometimes use two canes.

Being on your feet for a long time, and walking on the typical cement floors used in all malls, shopping centers and large department stores today will very likely cause pain and inflammation to set in before you have been shopping for very long. If I have a choice between an electric cart and suffering a flare-up when I get home, I favor the electric cart.

These floors may look like tile floors, wooden floors, stained floors, textured floors, beautifully painted and decoratively designed floors, but floors in most all modern day stores and some homes are made of concrete that has been stained, polished and/or given an application of a coating or overlay. If you have any kind rheumatic pain, this type of floor surface will definitely cause body fatigue in the form of foot, leg, neck and low back pain.

There are people who will not use an electric cart when they are shopping; they think electric carts are only for people on crutches or people with oxygen tanks. Yet these same people will lean on a shopping cart and tolerate great pain (very dangerous; but we have all done it); then go home and suffer a flare-up caused by their day of shopping.

CHANGES IN THE HOME AND WORK ENVIRONMENT

Changes in the home and workplace can help in many ways by making it easier to accomplish daily tasks without aggravating our fibromyalgia symptoms.

MAKING THE KITCHEN AND BATH AREAS USER-FRIENDLY

As a Kitchen and Bath Design Specialist, I understand how significantly a dysfunctional kitchen and bath can possibly affect the homemaker more than most areas of the home.

I have included a few tips on creating a user-friendly kitchen and bath area that may be of help to you.

IN THE BATH, of course the concern is for safety as well as convenience.

You may wish to discuss with a professional bath designer or an occupational therapy practitioner how your bath can be made more convenient and safe (based on your personal needs). Below are a few suggestions that you may find helpful:

- Consider using flooring that has a slip-resistant surface, especially for use around "water areas" such as the bath and shower.

- Be sure all areas of the bathroom have good lighting

- towel bars should be accessible to the bath and shower without having to take steps to gain access to a towel.

- There should be a sufficient amount of small shelves accessible within all bathing areas; making it easy to access various toiletries.

- An arched sink faucet with ergonomic handles that are easy to use can be very beneficial; especially for those who cannot wash their hair in the shower due to problems with their balance.

- Ergonomic toilets have slightly higher seats to accommodate those who have problems with pain when they get up from a sitting position.

- You may also benefit from choosing cabinetry that has "self-closing" drawers.

- Be sure there are electrical outlets not only around the sink area, but also close to the toilet area and any other areas where they may be needed.

- In the shower, you could consider a showerhead that comes with a separate handheld shower spray whose line attaches to the wall; this is especially useful for anyone who finds it safer to shower while sitting down.

- There are many safety tools that you can consider such as grab bars and shower seats.

  Be sure a qualified contractor (very important) installs the addition of any safety equipment such as grab bars, that you may wish to use within the bathing areas.

IN THE KITCHEN, many moderate changes can make your kitchen much easier to use. These changes include such things as:

- Flooring for the kitchen that is easier on the feet and legs.

  Flooring made of "bouncier materials" such as wood, cork or rubber do not put stress on your body like most tile floors do.

- Replacing stationary base cabinet shelves with shelves that roll out; thus reducing the pain of stooping down and reaching back to retrieve objects on the back of the shelf.

- At the kitchen sink, a handheld sprayer can be very helpful.

- The type of water faucets that you use can make a big difference. The arch-shaped, free moving, water faucets are often more convenient for many uses in the kitchen.

- New handles for the kitchen cabinets that are easier to grasp.

- Choose faucets that have ergonomic handles, making them easier to grasp.

- You can check your local home remodeling center to see what accessories and add-ons they may have that can be added to your present cabinetry.

IN THE WORKPLACE, some companies will provide a consultant to help your work space to become more ergonomic. If not, you can benefit from seeking advice from an occupational therapist.

Below are a few suggestions:

- If you stand a great deal of the time, make sure you have:

  ▪ high-quality, comfortable shoes

  ▪ A cushioned floor pad in the general area where you will be standing the most

  ▪ Access to seating for occasional breaks

- **If you sit most of the day,** invest in a high-quality ergonomic chair and some type of footrest.

- If you spend a lot of time on the phone, maybe you should consider using a type of headset.

FINDING SPACE FOR ACCESSIBLE PANTRIES

Anyone dealing with chronic pain should avoid making trips up and down steps if possible.

If the addition of a pantry would prevent daily trips to the basement, you may wish to add a pantry closer to the kitchen area.

You can have a contractor survey the situation to see if there are some possible solutions for you. Although the average pantry shelves are about twelve inches deep, pantry shelves can be as shallow as 4 to 6 inches deep and still be very useful.

If you have a bare wall that can accommodate a pantry, then you are in luck. Pantries can be located in dining rooms, kitchens, hallways, behind doors and even under staircases if fire codes in your area allow.

The important thing is to keep them shallow. Any depth shelves from 6 inches to 12 inches would be perfect for ease-of-use. This allows easy access to items you need without digging for them.

For example:

- If you have an exceptionally deep pantry closet area, you could make it more accessible by using 12 inch deep shelves inside the closet and then add additional wire shelving attached to the back of the pantry door.

- Shallow pantries can be set into the space between existing wall studs. They need only to protrude out slightly to accommodate a door frame and door.

- If you have limited space for a pantry, you can purchase "fold-out pantries that are about the size of a refrigerator". These pantries can be purchased in many finishes to match your present kitchen cabinetry.

PANTRIES MADE FROM WALL CABINETS

Stock cabinets can be used in many ways besides those they are designed for.

Wall cabinets can be used to create beautiful pantries; they can be as low as chair rail height or made to reach completely to the ceiling if you so wish.

- If you have a bare wall area, a contractor can easily make a twelve-inch deep pantry across the bare wall without the involvement of major construction by using wall cabinets.

  This can be done by making a footer under a wall cabinet and securing the cabinet to the base of the wall. You can then add more wall cabinets above this first cabinet to the height you wish your pantry to be. These pantries can be as low as chair rail height or as high as you wish.

  This idea works especially well in older homes that have very little cabinet space in the kitchen area.

Wall cabinets can also be used to easily create a beautiful "buffet and hutch" affect.

- To create a "buffet and hutch" look, your contractor can install any number of 27 inch to 33 inch high wall cabinets to the base of the wall to use as your "buffet" cabinet by making a simple footer for along the base of each cabinet and securing them to the wall.

- For the "hutch", wall cabinets can then be installed on the wall about 14 to18 inches above the *buffet* cabinet.

- If you wish to have a more decorative finish, you can have your contractor to replace the inset section on the upper cabinet doors with something like: glass, "bubble class", fitted curtains, stained-glass etc.

- Now all that is left to do is to choose the countertop material that you wish to use for on top of the "buffet" cabinet(s) and your buffet and hutch is completed.

  You can use this same idea (with or without the "hutch") across one side of your dining room or breakfast nook. Wall cabinets come in various heights and widths to accommodate the design you wish to make.

THE KITCHEN WORK TRIANGLE

The kitchen work space is made up of three major work areas. These are the areas surrounding the sink, the refrigerator and the stove top; this is referred to as the Work Triangle.

Your most helpful objective in the kitchen is to organize the cabinet contents within the work triangle so that kitchen activities can flow smoothly.

- The sink area is for washing produce and meats and for general cleanup.

- The cooktop area is for cooking.

- The refrigerator area is for food storage.

Nothing must interfere with the traffic flow between these three work areas. There should be no cabinets, island, tables or anything to cause you to have to "walk around" them to get from one work area to the other (this is very important).

When a triangle is drawn between these three work stations, the sum total of its sides would be best to not exceed twenty one feet. The closer these work areas are to each other, the more efficient the kitchen will be as it will take less steps to prepare a meal.

There should also be a work space accessible to these three work areas to provide room for gathering ingredients and preparing foods. This could be countertop space, a table, kitchen cart etc.; just be sure that this work area does not obstruct the traffic flow between the three major work areas.

KITCHEN "EASY- ACCESS AREAS"

Within the three work area in your kitchen, there are drawers and cupboards that are easily accessed with the least amount of reaching or bending being involved. "This is your "Easy Access Area".

In the base cabinets, this is the first and second drawer of a bank of drawers or the top drawer and top shelf of a base cabinet.

In the wall cabinets, this easy access area is the bottom shelf and possibly the second shelf (according to your height).

You will find it a lot easier to accomplish your daily routine if you keep these "easy access areas" clear of things seldom used. You should only keep those tools, dishes, spices etc. that you are most apt to use on a daily basis

This will save you a tremendous amount of running back and forth, and it will be easier to find the tools that you need.

If you have enough countertop room, frequently used items can even be used in a decorative way by displaying them in decorative containers and placing them on the countertop or hanging them on the wall instead of being hidden inside cupboards.

This can free up more storage space in drawers and cabinets within the easy access area; but be sure this does not make the countertop too cluttered to work on.

If you are considering mounting some of these items on a wall or hanging them; be sure that they are hung securely and will be easily accessible without excessive stretching.

IDEAS FOR ENHANCING YOUR "EASY ACCESS" AREA

- Dry goods that are used most often can be stored in decorative jars and placed on the countertop.

- A container for kitchen tools can be kept in the work area for the tools most often used such as kitchen scissors, wooden spoons, whisks etc.

- A small wire basket kept near the cooktop (but not too close) can be handy for keeping items close at hand that you most often use when you are cooking.

"I personally keep four or five "most often used seasonings" in a small wire basket near the cooktop with small bottles of olive oil and vinegar behind the basket. Then behind these bottles I keep a tall tool container to hold four or five most often used tools such as whisks, spatulas etc. Then behind the container of tools I keep a couple of potholders hanging on the wall. This combination takes up very little room and is a great help to me."

This saves me from repeatedly reaching up into the cupboard for cooking oil, desperately digging through drawers for tools and continuous trips to the spice rack.

- A spice rack, if you have the room, can be easily hung on a wall or set up on a countertop.

My husband "tailor-made" mine to fit my spice needs. Everyone that sees this spice rack wants one for themselves. It has five shelves and hangs on the wall (I still need more room).

- Some cabinet manufacturers make drawer units that fit into the 18 inch space between the countertop and the wall cabinets. If you have the room for such drawers, this makes an excellent place for keeping tools or spices.

- Single drawer units that fit just under the wall cabinets will provide storage space and still leave a valuable workspace area below.

- "Appliance garages" that match your cabinets can "Park" your small appliances etc. out of sight. They can be located in corners or anywhere along the countertop that you may have need of them.

- You can purchase kits to make the "false drawer" in the front of your sink cabinet into a "tip out" for storing sponges, scrubbers etc. out of sight.

- You can have a contractor (or a husband that is handy with tools) to install sliding shelves inside your existing base cabinets in place of your stationary shelves.

You can purchase these base cabinet "slide out drawer units" already installed in new cabinets. For existing cabinets, kits can be purchased at most kitchen centers; be sure that they are sturdy enough to hold heavy weight loads without tipping forward.

These are a great help because without doing a lot of bending and reaching back, you can reach what is on the back of the shelf.

- Decorative containers that contain cookies, candy, dog biscuits etc. that have nothing to do with food and drink preparation, should be kept in the areas far away from the "easy access" area.

- A hot beverage area that consists of such things as: a coffee maker, suspended coffee cups, baskets of individually wrapped tea bags and/or hot chocolate packets etc. can be very handy, but should be located just outside the "easy access area".

All kitchens are different, and all needs are different; so you will have to choose what works best for you. Your main goal is to have your tools "close at hand" and to not create a cluttered workspace.

USER-FRIENDLY COOKING HINTS

Getting your kitchen into user-friendly condition may require time and help, but once you have succeeded, you will find it much easier to prepare meals without aggravating your symptoms.

- Treat yourself to a new set of user-friendly cookware in the kitchen. Look for cookware that is not too heavy to handle and feels balanced when you pick it up.

- Lightweight stainless steel mixing bowls are much easier to handle than heavy glass or ceramic mixing bowls; especially when lifting them in and out of cupboards.

  Do not assume that all stainless steel mixing bowls are going to be lightweight. If buying them over the Internet, beware, they could be much heavier than they look.

- Take advantage of all electrical appliances that can help you to do your work each day. Place ones that you will need on a regular basis in a location easily accessible to your work area or you probably will not use them.

- If you have a rolling kitchen utility cart; use it. Do not let it sit in a corner with things stacked on top of it. It should always be empty so it can actually be used in ways to make your life easier; such as:

  - Transporting ingredients and other items when preparing a meal or when baking

  - As an extra countertop during meal preparation

  - Transporting a pot of boiling water from the stove to the sink area

  - Transporting heavy groceries when putting groceries away

  - Carrying dishes and foods to and from the table.

- When in the market for a new kitchen stove, consider a solid ceramic stovetop. With this, you can avoid having to clean out spillover trays and having to reach back and clean out underneath burners. Be sure to have someone explain to you how to keep the ceramic stovetop clean before you buy it.

More Helpful Ideas for the Kitchen
- Go through your kitchen cupboards, closets, and pantry and

weed out those things that you never use, but just did not want to get rid of. (you can store these in more inaccessible places, pack them away for storage or give them away).

- Try to simplify your main working area as much as you possibly can.

- Remove from your work areas, and possibly from your kitchen, anything that you know is going to require more strength or stamina to use then you can deal with at this time. You can always store them away until such time as you feel the need for them.

- In your endeavor to simplify your work area, do not overlook your assortment of food storage containers.

  Replacing the ones that have lids that are painful to impossible to remove with ones that are user-friendly will make your work much easier. once you have these unusable items out of the way, you will have more space in your work area.

"My 4'9" mother-in-law is wheelchair-bound due to a heart problem and arthritis. I was helping her to redo her kitchen in a way that would give her easy access to the things that she needed most."

"It took us two different sessions to go through her storage containers. The first time I convinced her to let go of all the yellowed ones that she had not used for years and the many orphans whose lids had disappeared long ago."

"The second time around, I had her to open every remaining container herself to see if she could actually use it. In doing this, if she had to, she would turn the container over on its side and struggle to open it. I would then point out to her that had it contained food, it would now be all over her lap."

"By the time we were through, she had "very" few containers left. Then I replaced the unusable containers with stackable, disposable containers (with lids that were easily opened) in the sizes that she most often used; she was delighted."

- A great way to eliminate frequent oven cleaning is to use an aluminum oven liner to line the floor of the oven. Even if you have a self-cleaning oven, you will have to clean it less often using these.

- If you use a teakettle, the ones with lids on top are easier to refill than the ones that refill through a spring open spout that you have to hold open (very tiring on the hands). Just be sure the lid is on tightly after filling in order to avoid an accident.

- If it hurts your hands to use a dishcloth, there is a type of dishcloth that is called a "scrubber dishcloth" that is much easier to use. These have terrycloth on one side and a crocheted polyester mesh on the other.

  By placing the polyester mesh against the surface you are cleaning, the dishcloth easily glides over the surface; causing less pain. (Do not confuse these with "waffle weave" dishcloths)

- It is a good idea to always keep a supply of paper plates, bowls, plastic eating utensils and cups on hand. Sometimes even a dishwasher can be too much for you to deal with and these disposables are definitely good to have on hand. *(Do not microwave in plastic or foam; you do not want to add to your body the toxic chemicals that these give off when heated)*

- For easy cleanup when you are microwaving food; you can place your food on a dinner plate or bowl that is lined with a sheet of parchment paper.

- Stiff potholders may be difficult to use if you are experiencing pain in your hands. Replace these with flexible potholders such as ones made from silicon or ones that are made from very thick terrycloth. A flexible potholder will give you more control and save you from painful burns and spills.

HINTS AND ACCESSIBLE AIDS

I have included this short section on accessible aids because often persons who have fibromyalgia also have pain from other sources such as arthritis, tendinitis, bursitis etc.

- If you experience weakness and/or pain in your hands or

arms when you reach over to pick something up that is on the back of the kitchen counter, you can often use one arm to help the weaker arm. You can do this by bringing your one hand up to support the elbow of the reaching arm.

- Electronic jar openers are handy, but they do take up a lot of counter space. If you want to use one of these on your counter, it would probably be best to keep it outside of your immediate work area. (This type of jar opener cannot be used to open plastic jars).

- The Kuhn Rikon Gripper Jar Opener is not electric, it is a hand-held gadget that grips the lid and has an attached handle for you to turn. Ease-of-use may not measure up to that of the electric ones that sit on the countertop, but I give it a five star. This opener grips the lid, not the jar, so it can be used on plastic jars also.

- The "JarKey" by Brix is an excellent tool for using on vacuum sealed lids. It allows you to simply "pop" the seal.

- Another solution for tight lids are the "four-inch" round, flexible, rubber gripper pads. These are great for lids or anything that is hard to get a grip on, and they are economical enough to keep them in various areas of the house, garage or outdoor shed where you may need them. I even keep one in the glove box in my car. You can usually find packages of these gripper pads at most department stores and dollar stores.

- Some soda pop and water bottles can be very stubborn. If you stop to buy a soda pop or bottle of water when you're out and about; try to open the bottle as soon as you pay for it. If you cannot get it to budge, asked the cashier to open it for you. If you bought it in a machine, go inside the business that is responsible for the machine and asked the clerk to open it for you. A rubber gripper pad is the best solution for this.

CHAPTER 16
THE HOUSEWORK DILEMMA

Breaking your housework up into 2 to 3 minute increments will take the stress of housework to a much lower level

The reason I added these chapters on doing housework and laundry is because housework and laundry are not only a continuous concern to fibromyalgia patients, but are also a constant source of stress.

If being constantly behind on your housework is one of the sources of your stress; then avoiding this stress to the best of your ability would definitely be essential to your overall health.

Like a vicious cycle; an increase in stress decreases the amount of serotonin activity in your brain, and a decrease in serotonin turns around and increases your fibromyalgia symptoms; which, in turn, will give cause to increased stress.

Anyone can attest to the fact that anytime they are ill or excessively busy, it is reflected in their housework. And most everyone has had times when housework has gotten a little out of hand due to some reason or another and you would feel uncomfortable if company showed up at your front door, unannounced, right at that time.

But when you have an illness that causes constant pain and exhaustion, this happens more often than not.

The need for continuous housework does not go away, no matter what the circumstances; showing the old adage "You don't notice housework until it's not being done" to be very true.

Housework is a continuous an unavoidable concern for those who have any chronic illness such as fibromyalgia. It is not that they do not want a clean house, but that sometimes even the thought of cleaning house hurts.

GETTING STARTED

We all have our priorities in life, but when you live with an illness that affects every area of your life the way fibromyalgia does, you may find life less stressful by calmly rethinking just what these priorities truly are. Such decisions will definitely help you as you start making a dent in your housework woes.

You can begin by deciding what your priorities are for each room of your home. By this, I mean what would be "the most noticeable thing that stands out in each room" that would make that particular room look messy when undone or less messy when it is done?

Have you ever noticed that no matter how neatly kept a bedroom is, it will look messy until the bed has been made? Even though the bedroom is a little messy, as long as that bed is neatly made, it will not seem as disorderly.

Therefore, in the bedroom the number one priority would be making the bed each day; very simple yet very effective.

Most of these things that make a great difference in whether a room looks neat or not can be taken care of in less than 10 minutes; if maintained daily.

If you try to make sure that at least "these priorities" for each room of your home are tended to each day, you will feel better about yourself.

You may feel up to doing more in a days' time, but starting your day by doing the things that you have predetermined to be the best use of your time, will get you off to a good start on your day.

SIMPLIFYING

In this day and time, it would seem everyone is constantly battling clutter.

If you went as far back as the early 1900s, there was very little clutter. With today's technologies and mass production of everything imaginable, you have endless mail, greeting cards, seldom used gadgets, magazines, old toys, outdated and unusable electronic treasures, boxes wrappers etc.

Too often, instead of getting rid of the clutter we buy plastic tubs, fill them with our clutter, and start all over again.

Perhaps this is okay for a healthy individual, but stressful for anyone with physical limitations.

There are two very helpful rules of thumb to use when trying to simplify your home:

1. If it is garbage, or has garbage potential, pitch it. (Garbage potential means "you're not using it and would never replace it"). The less you have to clean and the less clutter you have, the less stress you will have to deal with.

2. If it is something you can no longer use or do because of your health, you can either give it away, pack it away or sell it.

MAKING HOUSEWORK LESS STRESSFUL

Breaking your housework up into 2 to 3 minute increments will take the stress of housework to a much lower level and you will be surprised at just how much can be accomplished in two or three serious minutes of work.

For timing yourself, you can choose from various timers that can either be worn about the neck, carried in a pocket or pinned to your clothing. You can also find apps that can be used for this purpose.

If you wear a timer about the neck; you can purchase straps with "breakaway clasps" in most sporting goods departments. This type of timer is effective, but it can get in the way when you bend down; so you could try pinning the timer to your clothing or carrying it in your pocket. (Remember to remove it when you take a nap)

The timer you choose should be small and have a repeat function so that once a measure of time has been chosen, all you have to do is click the button to repeatedly reactivate it. Make sure to read all the customer reviews on any timer before you choose it.

If you are cleaning in three minute increments, you can now set your timer for three minutes and then just click it before starting each project.

When you have a job to do that you are not looking forward to doing or just do not feel up to doing, it is so much easier to just set your timer for two or three minutes and know that when that alarm goes off, no matter how little you have done, "You Are Out of There"!

Another very important use of such a timer would be to time your inactive/active times. There are two basic rules to consider:

1. Maximum time to be active (one hour or as you feel capable)

2. Maximum time to be inactive (30 minutes).

Timing these active and inactive periods is much easier with the help of a timer. You can set such timers by the push of a button (like the snooze alarm on your clock).

Using the convenience of a timer, you can start digging your way out of your "housecleaning dilemma" three minutes at a time or even less.

You will be surprised at how much you can accomplish in the short periods of time. On good days you may be able to set your active time periods to be longer than on other days.

For those days when you're really feeling well and hope to get a lot accomplished, it is all too easy to forget about taking frequent rest periods. For this reason, it is a good idea to have a small timer either in your pocket or attached to your clothing.

By setting the timer to the time you designate (usually 30 or 40 minutes), you'll be assured of remembering to take your frequent rest periods.

When the timer goes off, set aside whatever you're doing and take a rest or just do something that can be done while sitting.

It is amazing how just a few minutes of being inactive "before" you "feel tired" is often enough to give you the needed strength to continue for another 45 minutes or so.

No matter how short or long you choose to have these active periods to be, remember to not be inactive for longer than 30 minutes.

CLEANING CADDIES

"How many times have you wanted to do a little work but by the time you gathered up the tools and cleaning products, you were already getting tired?"

There is a very simple solution to this dilemma. Using a container such as a small bucket or any sort of container that fits into your available space requirements, you can create a cleaning caddy made up of just the amount of tools necessary for many smaller jobs that you may feel like tackling.

These caddies should be kept small and filled with only a "few essentials" pertaining to what is practical for the area of the house it will be used in.

SUGGESTIONS FOR A CLEANING CADDY'S CONTENTS:

- A Spray bottle of child safe, antibacterial cleaner (half distilled vinegar/half water")
- Small Sponge
- Feather duster
- Small roll of paper towels

- Small whisk broom with an attached dustpan
- "Eraser sponge" for grunge
- Plastic shopping bags... the kind that you get at the grocery with little cut out holes for handles (you can poke several of these inside a plastic cup and place inside the caddy)

Whenever practical, you would also benefit from having a couple of areas throughout the home set up for quick access to some type of broom/dustpan combination and perhaps in some cases even a sponge mop. These can be kept out of sight, nestled just inside a closet, behind a door or anywhere they can be squeezed in unnoticed.

okay, now you are armed with a timer, the knowledge of how to use it to your advantage, and a well-stocked cleaning caddy located where you will need it most.

These caddies are so helpful, that you may want to make up several. You could keep one caddy in each bathroom and others in any other location throughout your home where you would want quick and easy access to your tools and supplies.

Now housework will not be the formidable task it once was. Being able to "chip away" at the smaller jobs, when you do not feel up to doing larger jobs, will make overall housework much easier to do.

*It is very important that you remember to toss tools back into the cleaning caddy after using them so they will be there the next time they are needed.

ADVANTAGES OF USING A "BETWEEN TASKS LIST"
Sometimes when you need a break from your routine, it is good to get your mind onto something else for a short time by creating a diversion from routine. This is where a list of alternate activities, already made up for you to choose from, comes in handy.

A "Between-Task list" is a list of short or easy tasks and activities that you can sandwich between lengthy activities in your daily routine; long, drawn out jobs can become tedious even if you do stop for breaks. This is when a "change of scenery" is needed.

These little "between job activities" are not necessarily jobs, they can be a variety of things from short jobs to relaxing activities. This list can be used over and over because it never becomes outdated. It is made up of three types of activities:

1. Easy jobs

2. Activities that relax you

3. Quickie jobs

1. EASY JOBS

These are usually easier tasks that cause very little physical stress; they can be sitting or standing jobs. While these jobs are not complicated or stressful, they are not necessarily short in duration.

They can range from washing the lettuce for dinner to sorting through that stack of magazines and discarding outdated ones, or whatever else you consider easy to do.

2. ACTIVITIES THAT RELAX

These activities are for when you feel yourself becoming tensed up. They can be short or long and the best ones are mind absorbing. This allows you to get your mind off the current work that you are doing.

The activities that you choose for on this list could be something like taking a walk, spending a few minutes on a type of mind puzzle, listening to music as you relax, or just simply spending some time with a pet.

You may not feel you need to make a listing of these activities, but when you are tired, your mind is tired. It helps to not have to think; just choose.

3. QUICKIE JOBS

this is a list that provides you with "quick" jobs you can do in between your regular activities.

How many times have you come upon something that would only take "a minute to do" and you put it off until "later" (such as wiping off the wall plate behind the electrical wall switches).

These jobs can be quickly done and this is the reason why they are often put off until later and can too easily build up into big "yucky" jobs.

If you wish, you could even go farther by marking which jobs could be done while sitting and which require being done while standing.

Using Your "Between" Tasks List

Using the lists that you made will make your pacing routine work better for you on a daily basis. They will provide you with ideas for a list of quick jobs that you can use effectively.

You can return to the original task "off and on" during the day if you wish to, rather than becoming stressed or exhausted by "sticking with it" to the end.

"The main idea is to keep a balance in your activities"

- Standing activities…Sitting activities
- Hard Activities…Easy activities
- Stressful Activities…Relaxing activities

Examples of things that could go on your lists:

- Any of the two or three minute increment jobs you listed for the bathroom, family room etc.

- Go through the growing stack of catalogs/or magazines and toss some outdated ones into the garbage.

- Clean out your purse.

- Clean a mirror. This can be any one of the many you have in your home.

- Shake out your front entry mat/back door entry mat.

- Sweep the front entry area/back door entry to your home.

- Go through your cleaning supplies and toss empty bottles and boxes into the garbage.

- Update your cleaning caddies.

- Change the light bulb over the range.

- Go through your mail and toss out the junk mail.

- Goes through your medicine cabinet and see if there are any outdated medicines that need to be tossed out.

- Go through your first-aid kit and see if it needs updated.

- Do a thorough cleaning of the lint filter in your dryer.

- Clean an annoying stain that you never seem to have the time to stop and clean.

- Refill your spray cleaner bottle(s).

- Wipe off small appliances in the kitchen.

- Clean the microwave interior.

- Wash off the refrigerator door.

- Check your "things for today" list.

- Clean out or organize a drawer.

- Tidy up the computer desk.

- Vacuum the cat condo.

- Put flea medicine on the dog (or cat).

- Shake or vacuum out the dog bed (and give it a light misting of white vinegar to minimize odor and kill fleas).

- Dust out one shelf of a bookcase.

- Rearrange one row of books in a bookcase.

- Go through the bathroom cabinets and throw away empty or long neglected bottles and aerosol cans.

- Tidy up the linen closet (nothing radical, just a tidy up).

- Dust a ceiling fan.

- Pay a bill.

- Empty the garbage in the bathroom.

- Empty the garbage in the kitchen.

- Put the plastic liner in a garbage can.

- Clean the birdcage.

- With a feather duster or vacuum, dust ceiling edges and corners.

- Take the mail to the mailbox.

- Pick up mail from mailbox

MAKING PACING WORK

Any time you start a project large or small, your number one priority that you want to keep in mind is pacing yourself.

When you are having a "good day", you may feel tempted to take advantage of this and start a big project. There is nothing wrong with starting a big project as long as you pace yourself.

- First, you must make yourself take rest periods "before" you are tired.

- Break the big job up into several smaller jobs that can be completed every so often.

- Make sure that the first part of a job is cleared away or stacked neatly out of the way before stopping or before tackling part two of the job.

By completing each part of the job and straightening up the work area before stopping, you will find that if you do suddenly have a relapse, you will not leave such a mess behind...only a small one, and you will not dread going back to it another day because of the mess.

- Make sure that as you pace yourself with rest periods, that you also balance your day by going from standing to sitting activities.

- After about an hour of being busy, stop for a snack or take a rest.. You will find that you will come back to the job, each time, refreshed and better able to think after a rest period.

- If you are careful to pace yourself, you will develop an awareness of those times when you need to stop for rest and you will have a much better chance of not feeling "wiped out" when you are done.

The idea of pacing yourself can be incorporated into all your daily activities and hobbies so you do not have to give up things that you love to do; you just have to learn to break tasks up into smaller parts.

Quotable Quotes

I hate housework!
You make the beds,
You do the dishes and
Six months later you have
To start all over again.

Joan Rivers

......
Housework can't kill you,
Why take the chance?

Phyllis Diller

My theory on housework is,
If the item doesn't multiply,
Smell, catch fire, or block
The refrigerator door let it be.
No one else cares.
Why should you?

Erma Bombeck

CHAPTER 17
HOUSECLEANING THREE MINUTES AT A TIME

"How can I do housework when I suffer with pain and fatigue?"

Housework can be very challenging for those who have fibromyalgia. Not only do you not feel good, but sometimes, during times of having flare-ups or physical or emotional stress, you find yourself too exhausted or in too much pain to even do light housework. These kinds of setbacks cause you to get even further behind in your housework.

When we talk about cleaning house in this section on housekeeping, keep in mind that everyone who has fibromyalgia is different. If your symptoms are a mere stiffness and tiredness, count yourself fortunate and realize that the majority of fellow sufferers endure extreme chronic pain and fatigue.

For some people, fibromyalgia is a very debilitating illness that they have had over a long length of time and it is going to take a lot of time and determination for them to start seeing a light at the end of the tunnel.

A flare-up that lasts for three or four days could leave you with quite a housecleaning problem if you factor in three children and a husband to the picture.

No one plans to let housecleaning problems get out of hand; but it can happen when dealing with pain and fatigue on a daily basis.

Then when you try to catch up, you have to be very careful not to push yourself so hard that you could suffer another flare up.

When you do housework in timed sessions, it makes it possible for you to carry out your cleaning routine in such a way as to not aggravate your symptoms. Timed cleaning sessions could be as short as one minute to an average of five minutes; it is all up to you.

Be good to yourself and use any tools that you find helpful. This could be anything from telescoping dusters or telescoping grabbers to well-made step stools.

A word of caution about using a stepstool; many people with fibromyalgia have balance related problems so you should put a lot of thought into your choice of a stepstool.

Step stools that have a grab bar curved over top of the stool for you to grab onto in case you lose your balance can be very helpful. Be sure there are rubber caps on the feet made of a grabby type of rubber so the stool will not slide while you are standing on it.

Another feature you may want to consider is how easy it is to open and close the stepstool.

Below you will find a few suggestions on how you can use the idea of cleaning in timed sessions. As mentioned earlier you can adjust the timed sessions to the length of time that you feel you can handle; not everyone is at the same activity level.

Remember, the good thing about using timed sessions is that they do not have to be accomplished all at one time; each step can be accomplished at various times throughout the day.

Before we start talking about cleaning, please consider this: it is best for anyone who has fibromyalgia to avoid chemical cleaners. Distilled vinegar has excellent antibacterial properties and is better in some cases of mildew, than bleach. A spray bottle containing a mixture of half water and half distilled vinegar makes a very good all-purpose cleaner.

For soap scum, just add a few drops of Castile soap to the bottle of water/vinegar. As with all cleaning products, it is necessary to provide adequate ventilation when using vinegar for cleaning.

CLEANING A BATHROOM IN TIMED SESSIONS

- Grab all the dirty clothes, towels etc. and toss them into a hamper: (Three minutes)

- Toss any garbage into the trash container: (Three minutes)

- Pick up a rug; fluff it, and put it back down: (Two minutes)

- Pick up any clutter off the countertop and put it away: (Three minutes)

- Spray the bathroom countertop**, mirror and surrounding areas with all-purpose cleaner (vinegar/water); then wipe them down with paper towels: (Three minutes) (**do not use vinegar on marble countertops)

- Sweep bathroom floor with a dust mop or electric broom: (Three minutes)

- Spray shower door, with all-purpose cleaner (vinegar/water plus a few drops of Castile soap). Wipe the shower door down with paper towels or sponge: (Four minutes)

- Spray the entire outside of the toilet with full strength vinegar or peroxide. Wipe it down with paper towels: (Four Minutes)*be sure there is adequate ventilation.

- Spray the bathroom window with all-purpose cleaner or window cleaner and wipe it down with paper towels or sponge. (Three minutes)

- Pour one or 2 cups distilled vinegar into the toilet bowl. Brush around the bowl and up under the rim. Put the lid down and place a designated object on top of the lid so others will know it has cleaner in it and so you will not forget to come back to it.

Let the vinegar set while you do something else. Come back 10 or 15 minutes later to brush and flush: (You can add a couple tablespoons of baking soda to the toilet bowl just before you brush): (Three minutes)

- Run hot water over a sponge mop and squeeze it out to prepare it for use. Pour distilled vinegar/water mix over mop and squeeze out excess.

Spray the bathroom floor with distilled vinegar/water. (If you have carpeting, check for color fastness) Quickly run the sponge mop the floor and rinse out the mop. There is no need to rinse floor, because you did not use a soapy cleaner: (Three minutes)

- To wash walls; using a dampened sponge mop, spray the sponge mop with appropriate wall cleaner mixture and wipe walls down (rinsing mop and reapplying mixture as needed). (Five minutes
(for wallpapers and special wall finishes, follow manufacturer's suggested cleaning instructions.)

(For wood paneling, Clean wood paneling and door facings with a solution of 3 tablespoons oil, such as olive oil, ½ cup white vinegar, 2 tablespoons lemon concentrate and 2 cups of warm water.)

SUGGESTIONS FOR CLEANING THE FAMILY ROOM IN THREE MINUTE SESSIONS

If toys are a problem then you could enlist the help of the owners of the toys to remove them before you clean.

Even two-year-olds are happy to help by dropping toys into a box. Just remember, most children do not like to work alone; find work to do in the same room that they are working in; they like to work "with you" not alone.

You can even try making this and any other work your helpers do into a game and have a cookies and milk "party" or watch a video etc. at the end of the cleanup.

Giving children responsibilities when they are small and reinforcing their efforts with lots of praise will make your job much easier in the future.

Below are a few suggestions to help you get started cleaning the family recreation area in timed sessions: some may have to be repeated in several sessions, but that's okay…this is just an example of how to break cleaning into short periods of time so you can clean without over exerting yourself.

- For convenience, you can place the two containers beside each other on chairs.
  One basket will be for things that belong in this room but are out of place.
  The other basket will be for things that belong in other rooms.

- Remove from the floor, chairs, tables and shelves: anything that belongs in other rooms. Place these items into the proper container to distribute later.

- Straighten magazines or books and place them in a neat stack (do not sort at this time).

- Brush anything that is under the couch cushions out onto the floor

- Brush off couch cushions and fluff the pillows.

- Rather than having to bend down repeatedly, use a broom to gather any remaining toys, litter etc. left on the floor into a central area of the room near the two baskets.

- Place a garbage can, a dust pan and a chair next to the small mound of toys, litter etc.

- Now you can sit down and drop everything into its appropriate basket or into the garbage can and use the dustpan to finish up.

- You can distribute the contents of the containers later. When you empty these containers, this also can be done in three minute increments. (If small children are involved, use your imagination and their help for returning toys and other items to other rooms. They can make believe they are making deliveries, or even compete to see who can make the delivery faster than the other)

*A Note About Vacuuming

- If your present vacuum sweeper is difficult for you to handle, you may want to invest in one that is lighter or easier for you to use.

- Never buy a vacuum cleaner without trying it out first or making sure that you can return it if it is too difficult for you to use.

- Read all the reviews on the product before making any final buying decisions.

- Tank type vacuum sweepers are easier for some people because the wand is lightweight; making it easier to handle.

- Self-propelled sweepers can be helpful, but remember to only go forward with them; they are usually heavy and pulling back on them would be physically stressful.

- Whatever type of vacuum you get, you may find it easier and less stressful to keep the wand or vacuum near to you as you sweep. If you have it close to you, you can walk it forward and walk it backwards rather than stretching your arms out and pulling back.

- Vacuuming is one job that, if possible, you may wish to ask help with; especially with the moving of heavy couches and chairs.

SUGGESTIONS FOR USING THREE MINUTE TASKS TO CLEAN A KITCHEN

- Take a plastic shopping bag and use it to quickly go around and pick up any litter on tables or counters from snacks etc.

- If there are dishes sitting in the dishpan, take them out and fill the dishpan with hot sudsy water.

- Use a plastic mesh scour pad under running hot water to remove any debris on plates, bowls etc. before placing them into the hot sudsy water. Let them sit in the hot soapy water until they have soaked for about five minutes; making them easier to wash.

- Now you can wash the dishes or put them into the dishwasher and you can use the warm sudsy water for cleaning countertops etc. instead of toxic smelling chemicals (adding a cup of vinegar to the dishwater changes it into an antibacterial cleaner, but it will also reduce the sudsy slipperiness of the dishwater.)

- Wipe the refrigerator door using the warm dishwater.

- Run a sponge or dishcloth over the stove top and the oven door.

- Wipe the microwave door and any other small appliances.

- Wipe out the interior of the microwave oven. If there is food stuck to the walls and ceiling of the microwave, wet two paper towels (very wet) and place them onto the microwave plate. "Cook" the wet paper towels for a minute and let them set there to cool while you do something else. When you come back, the towels will be cooled and the food on the microwave walls and ceiling will wipe off easily.

- Take the microwave removable glass turntable over to the dishpan; wash and dry it before returning it to the microwave.

- Wipe off countertops and tabletops.

- Wipe the sink and water spigots with an "eraser sponge" and rinse.

SUGGESTIONS FOR CLEANING THE REFRIGERATOR IN THREE MINUTE INCREMENTS

One way to do this is to pick a day that you have no pressing jobs to do. You can spend the day cleaning your refrigerator at your leisure.

Have sufficient leftovers or something ready-made for dinner that you can just pop into the oven so you can make this a day of paper plates and no cooking.

Depending on how you want to do it, you can cut the refrigerator cleaning into short 3-minute breaks taken throughout your day's routine, or you could put in a movie and pause it every so often to spend two or three minutes working on your "fridge".

You do not have to be overly concerned with keeping the foods cold because you will only have the refrigerator door open three minutes or less at a time.

- Pull a garbage can and a chair close to the refrigerator area.

- At this time, you are not going to be concerned with leftovers that are in dishes that would have to be washed. You are only going to toss into the garbage such things as: empty containers, outdated containers, anonymous things lurking in foil or plastic bags and vegetables and fruits that have seen better days etc.

- Leftovers: Each time you have a few minutes to spend on the fridge, take out one container that has "been there too long" and dump the contents into the garbage. Fill the container with water and let it set in the sink to soak. Continue throughout the day until all such containers are emptied.

- If there is anything else left in the refrigerator that you wish to discard, do it at this time.

- Wash any glass shelves…one per session

- Wash any wire shelving…one per session

- Wash out one drawer per session

- Clean out any "cubbies"…one per session

- Wash the refrigerator walls…one wall per session

- Wash the floor of the refrigerator

- Last but not least, wash the empty food containers that you left sitting in the sink.

If you did not wish to do this entire project in one day, it can also be easily spread out over several days; it is completely up to you.

USING NATURAL CLEANERS IN PLACE OF DANGEROUS CHEMICALS

You should try to eliminate as many chemicals from your life as possible; especially when you have a health problem such as fibromyalgia.

- For an all-purpose cleaner, you can use distilled vinegar and water (mixed half and half) in a spray bottle. This makes a very good all-purpose cleaner that is also an excellent antibacterial cleaner. (Add a few drops of Castile soap to the mixture for hard grime such as soap scum)

- Use the vinegar full strength for stronger antibacterial cleaning. But as with all cleaners, be sure to supply adequate ventilation; just because it is natural does not mean it is safe to use it in a closed in space. (*Do not use vinegar on marble countertops)

- If you have trouble finding a comfortable sprayer to use for housecleaning purposes, you can also check the lawn and garden department for spray bottles that may be more user-friendly to use. Test the trigger on the sprayer to see if it is easily used when squeezed repeatedly.

CLEANING HINTS USING DISTILLED VINEGAR

- If you go online, you will find an abundance of suggested uses for vinegar. It is truly a multipurpose liquid.

- Clean wood paneling and door facings with a solution of 3 tablespoons oil (such as olive oil), ½ cup white vinegar, 2 tablespoons lemon concentrate and 2 cups of warm water.

- A clean sponge mop can make cleaning walls much quicker and will reduce the amount of stretching needed for the job. For special wall treatments and wallpaper, be sure to follow manufacturer's instructions for cleaning.

- Do not use vinegar on marble countertops

- You can make your own Soft Scrubber cleaner by combining ¼ cup baking soda, 1 tablespoon liquid Castile soap (or liquid dish detergent), and 1 teaspoon distilled vinegar.
                                OR
  Use an "eraser sponge" in place of soft scrubbers...for less mess

- Deodorizing a drain: pour 1 cup of baking soda into drain, add 1 cup "warm" (Not boiling) white vinegar. Pour the vinegar into the drain and let it sit for 10 or 15 minutes. Flush with hot tap water.

- Deodorizing and cleaning the microwave of hardened food deposits can be easily done by placing a microwave safe bowl containing 1 cup vinegar and ½ cup water into the microwave and bringing it to a boil.

Do not open the door for about three minutes. Do not discard the vinegar, save it to use in your spray cleaner bottle or one of the other many uses you can find for vinegar.

- In the laundry, use ¼ cup to ½ cup distilled vinegar in the last rinse. This softens clothes, reduces static cling and prevents yellowing. *I have used this method for over three years; I no longer need to use the smelly dryer sheets.*

  Another way to help reduce odors and soften clothes, try adding ¼ cup baking soda to your wash.

- Kill fleas by spraying full strength white vinegar into areas where you suspect your four-legged friends may transport them; places like the dog's bed, the cats condo etc.

  Do Not spray full strength vinegar onto your pets. Check with your veterinarian about whether you can safely use a very diluted vinegar/water to spray onto pets. (Vinegar sprayed into a pets eyes could cause blindness) Do Not Use On Cats.

Found in Emily Thacker's book "Vinegar Anniversary Book":

"The Yale New Haven Hospital uses distilled vinegar as a hospital disinfectant. When after-surgery-eye infections came a problem, their Department of Bacteriology solved it with vinegar."

…………………………………..

"The American Academy of Otolaryngology's

doctors who specialize in treating infections
like swimmer's ear now recommends using
a vinegar mixture as an antibacterial
preventative."

Using distilled vinegar is definitely a good substitute for cleaners made with toxic chemicals that could be hazardous to the health of anyone who has any kind of an autoimmune dysfunction.

When using vinegar be sure to follow the same safety rules as with other cleaners and provide adequate ventilation.

I'd rather attempt to do
Something great and fail
Than to attempt to do
Nothing and succeed

Robert S. Schuller
****

What you do today
Can improve all
Your tomorrows

Ralph Marston

CHAPTER 18
LAUNDRY HINTS

Tips for making laundry chores easier

Laundry can be a difficult chore to cope with. Not only does the laundry have to be constantly washed, but after you wash it and dry it you have to turn around and fold it up and put it away again.

You should not push yourself to do things the way you did them pre-fibromyalgia. You want to do things the least painful way you can, in order to achieve the results with which you can personally feel comfortable.

With laundry, as with other housework, you will find it necessary to see what your true priorities really are and begin there.

- So your clothes and linens look like your five-year-old folded them (and maybe they did). The main thing is that the clothes are clean and out of sight.

- You can drop sheets, blankets etc. into a basket placed on a closet shelf. They can be folded, rolled, or who cares how; they are clean and put away and that is all that matters. Congratulate yourself.

- The best way to avoid having to fold sheets and blankets is to take the sheets off the bed; wash and dry them and put them right back on the bed.

- When you hang a shirt on a hanger, you do not have to button it up. If you find buttoning a shirt too painful to do, care enough about yourself to be content that you did your best.

- When you put a shirt on the hanger, it is on a hanger where it should be; before it's worn, you can use a fabric steamer or you can mist it with water and iron it. You will find this to be much easier because you are not doing a lot of laundry and ironing at one time when you do it this way.

- Another tip: If you do have to iron; using a "barstool" to sit on while you iron may help take the stress off of your back and hips as you iron.

- Another quick trick for clothes (depending on the material they are made from) is to just spray them with a good misting of water and toss them into the dryer just before you wear them. Dry them for just a few minutes; remove immediately from the dryer and hang them or straighten them out.

- Many people find it much easier to take the wrinkles out of clothing using either a portable or a stationary fabric steamer for touchups instead of an iron.

General Laundry Hints
- You may wish to make your wash loads a little on the smaller side. This way you will not have as much trouble handling the wet clothes; the clothes will dry looking nicer and possibly less wrinkled (requiring less work) and you will not have as many clothes to put away at one time.

- Keep a wrist support in your laundry area to use when handling heavier clothes. You will want a wrist support that is supportive yet allows for more flexibility when you are working.

- Teach your children to wash and fold their own clothes. There is no reason any child over three years old cannot be taught to at least help you fold their clothes.

  You may have to adjust your attitude about what is acceptable or you could lose your helper, but allowing them to take part in doing their own laundry will assure you that as a child grows older they will be able to wash and fold their own clothes every bit as well as you can.

- Consider purchasing a front loading washer and dryer when you are in the market for a new laundry set (or a top-loader that has no agitator to contend with). Some have the option of a base drawer that they can be placed upon. This reduces your need for bending and stretching significantly.

- If you have a lot of back pain, and you have a top loading washer, you may find it easier to drop clean wet clothes into a clothes basket on the floor next to you; then scoot this basket over to the dryer.

- You may find it helpful to place a chair in front of your front loading dryer to sit on as you toss the clothes into the dryer and then again when you remove them from the dryer.

- If your laundry is on the same floor as the bedrooms, you can use a "wheeled shopping caddy" or wheeled laundry cart to transfer clothes from the dryer to the bedrooms.

- An easier way to transport soiled clothing to the washer is to use net or cotton laundry bags. These can be dragged to the washer using the ropes that are used to tie them shut. You may find it somewhat easier to handle these laundry bags than trying to carry a heavy load of clothing using a laundry basket.

IF YOU HAVE A BASEMENT LAUNDRY AND PUTTING THE LAUNDRY ON A MORE ACCESSIBLE FLOOR IS NOT IN YOUR FUTURE, YOU MAY FIND SOME OF THESE SOLUTIONS HELPFUL:

- If you must carry clothes up the stairs yourself, make sure the laundry baskets are smaller so they are easier and lighter to handle.

- Sort clean laundry into separate baskets for each person and let their owners carry their individual baskets upstairs (use small baskets for smaller children).

- Try to only do one wash a day unless you intend to spend most of that day in the basement. This reduces the risk of injury caused by going up and down stairs repeatedly.

You can set up a routine around the various timing cycles of the washer and dryer. This allows you to relax while the clothes wash, if you need to.

- Try keeping your wash loads on the smaller side when doing laundry. Not only do you put stress on your arms when trying to pull clothes out of a washer that is "packed tightly", but clothes come out more wrinkled when the wash load is larger.
It can also be more physically stressful to fold a really big load of clothes up all at one time..

- If you keep your wash loads a little on the small side, you will spend a shorter time when both removing clothes from the dryer and putting the dry clothes away.

- This whole process will not usually take more than 15 minutes. You could then have about 30 to 45 minutes to yourself before you have to repeat the process again.

RELOCATING THE LAUNDRY

One of the challenges many of us must deal with is the location of

THE FIBROMYALGIA CHALLENGE

the laundry.

Too often, the laundry is located in the basement. This presents us with the problem of traveling up and down the stairs more than we should. This could cause inflammation, pain and possible injury.

If you experience pain in your hip (which is common with fibromyalgia), there is a need for extra caution when you're going up and down stairs to prevent falls.

LOCATION OF THE LAUNDRY IS IMPORTANT
While a one-story ranch house would be the ideal, not all homes are designed with disability issues in mind. Many homes have an upstairs, a downstairs and possibly a basement. The ideal location of the laundry would be on the same floor where most of this soiled laundry originates but, unfortunately, that is not always possible.

Your contractor can often adapt something like a closet area to become the new home for your washer and dryer but many things have to be considered before choosing the proper location.

If you do not have room for your washer and dryer where you need it, you may want to consider replacing your washer and dryer with a washer/dryer combination unit that takes up the place of only one machine.

CHOOSING LAUNDRY APPLIANCES FOR LIMITED SPACES
There are three obvious choices for limited spaces. Make sure, before you make a decision to purchase any of these, that you check online for reviews and possibly "YouTube.com" for a video of their use.

1. There is the **"Combo Washer/Dryer"**, which is one machine that will both wash and dry clothes in the same unit. The cost for this unit is comparable to the cost of a washer and dryer set.

The advantages in using a combination washer/dryer unit are four-fold:

- First you have the advantage of only needing room for the one unit.

- Second, because you will only need room for one unit, it will be much easier to find a place for it closer to the bedroom area of your home.

- Third, some of these machines do not have to be vented to the outside; thus making it easier to find a suitable location for them.

- The fourth advantage is that you will not have to bother with lifting heavy, wet clothes from the washer to the dryer because the clothes will wash and dry in the same machine.

- One of the only drawbacks would be that these machines take almost twice as long, from start to finish, to do a wash. (But it does eliminate the need to handle heavy wet clothing.)

2. The **"Stackable Units"** are front loading and stack one on top of the other.

These are usually "regular-sized" machines, but of course they only take up the footprint of one machine.

The one thing you will want to consider with this choice would be whether you want to be lifting heavy wet clothes into an overhead dryer.

3. The **"Laundry Center"** (only about 27 inches wide) is not to be confused with "stackable units".

The **"laundry center"** is one unit, with the dryer over the washer. This unit takes up very little space, but be sure to check the capacity. For most of these units, just one king sized sheet may be more than you can wash in one load.

As with the stackable units though, you will also want to consider whether you want to be lifting heavy wet clothes into an overhead dryer.

Ideas Your Contractor May Suggest
- If you have a porch off your kitchen, 7 to 10 feet of this porch could possibly be enclosed for a laundry room.

- A laundry/closet could be added along the wall of the dining room or any other room. You can then add sliding or folding doors to blend well into your wall treatment. No one would ever guess the closet to be a "laundry room".

- A spare bedroom can become a laundry/bedroom:

A contractor could cut a small section out of a spare bedroom and make a laundry area that opens out into a hallway.

Be sure to check with a reputable contractor before making any such decisions. They will be able to supply you with the best possible choices.

The way to get started

Is to quit talking

And begin doing-

Walt Disney

****

Yesterday is not

Ours to recover,

But tomorrow is

Ours to win or lose

Lyndon B. Johnson

CHAPTER 19
FAMILY AND HOLIDAYS

The holiday seasons, starting with Thanksgiving and all the way through to the New Year's celebration, are the busiest, most family oriented times of the year in North America.

As with most traditional holiday seasons, wherever you live, the beauty of the holiday is wrapped up in events of the past as well as the present.

Holidays inevitably involve such things as: cooking, family visits, shopping, decorating, and invitations to various holiday events.

Unfortunately, the exhaustion and overwhelming feelings that can accompany them can be devastating to someone dealing with chronic pain and exhaustion.

Planning ahead for how you intend to celebrate a holiday season will reduce the stress and allow you to enjoy the festivities rather than being overcome by too much holiday preparation.

Take time to rethink your priorities. Perhaps this year you can make some changes in the way you celebrate the season that will allow you to enjoy the festivities without severe consequences.

REDUCING PHYSICAL AND MENTAL HOLIDAY STRESS

- If preparations for a big family dinner is too stressful, consider eating out at a restaurant.

- Many restaurants and some grocers offer a precooked holiday meal that can be delivered to your home the day before the holiday occasion (some require you to pick up your order yourself). All you have to do is refrigerate the dinner in the provided containers and reheat it the next day.

- If you will be expecting guests for dinner, you could ask each guest to bring either a desert or something to add to the meal/or both if they wish to. Make sure to ask them to keep you advised as to what they are bringing or you may end up with many of the same dish. A couple of versions of the same dish may be interesting, but there are limitations on just how many are practical.

- Instead of overextending your energies, you could consider buying deli made, bakery fresh, frozen or precooked desserts and dishes instead of expending your energies on these preparations. (*Ask if there is an ingredients list available to have on hand for guests who may have food allergies or sensitivities)

- In order to allow yourself time to relax and enjoy your guests, you could consider using disposable tablecloths, eating utensils, plates and cups. Even though you have a dishwasher, it will likely be full of serving and baking dishes.

- Using disposable plastic storage containers and plastic zipper bags, of various sizes for leftovers will save on having to repeatedly wash dishes.

- To help out on those extra busy days, it is good to keep lots of frozen, or easily prepared, meals and snacks on hand to help you out when needed.

- If decorating for the holiday has always been important to you, you may want to approach it in a different way in order to make it less stressful. You could ask for volunteers to put up the decorations for you.

- You may ask for volunteers to clean your house before the festivities or you may wish to enlist the services of a cleaning agency.

- You may consider putting out fewer holiday decorations than before. One or two large items are easier to deal with than scads of smaller ones.

- It may be easier to let someone else take on the responsibilities of the family get together this year and offer them your assistance if needed.

- You may wish to explain to family members, ahead of time, that you have to now be careful to not over expend your energies.

    Explain that there may be times when you have to disappear for a few minutes to rest, in order to prevent an increase in the intensity of your symptoms.

It is important for you to plan months in advance for the holiday festivities so you are not deprived of enjoying these joyous holidays and times of celebration with your family.

Do this planning when your mind is at its clearest and write everything down so you will have a working plan available just in case you are suddenly beset with a "down time" with lots of fibro fog.

So choose what you want to do, plan how you will do it, and enjoy your holiday.

SHARING THE WORK
Getting together with other people and making a day of doing various kinds of holiday preparations at each person's home can be very beneficial for everyone involved.

When three or more work together, work goes faster and it makes the season more festive to be sharing it with other people.

Although this is a great way to spend time with friends and to try new ideas, be sure to explain, before arrangements are made for a get-together, that having fibromyalgia places limits on your activities.

This "sharing-the-work" concept can be used in all areas of holiday preparations such as housecleaning, decorating, giftwrapping, costume making etc. It is always easier to work with someone than alone.

The more people involved in a project, the more ingenious ideas on how to get things done in a more efficient way.

Another thing you will find great about doing things with a group is that each person will have different areas in which they are best. This will make the work flow much easier for everybody and much more will be accomplished in much less time.

If you always enjoyed doing lots of baking, candy making etc. you may consider this "sharing" approach for these projects also.

Call around and see if there is a group already doing this that you could join, or call people that you know who do a variety of the same things that you enjoy doing and see if they would be interested in starting such a group activity.

If you do choose to work with a group, be sure to explain that you have to pace your activities by taking short breaks so the project does not become too overwhelming.

ALTERNATIVE IDEAS FOR PREPARING HOLIDAY BAKED GOODS

There are many ways to approach this part of the festivities:

- Check ehow.com or other such online sites for suggestions on freezing cakes, pies, cookies, cookie dough etc. several months ahead.

- Use a local bakery's services for cookies, cakes and pies.

- Purchase boxed baking mixes and refrigerated cookie dough.

- Buy your pies ready to bake or prebaked.

- Buy piecrusts in the dairy case, frozen, or ready-made.

HOLIDAY PRESSURE FROM FRIENDS AND FAMILY

Remember that holidays are supposed to be something enjoyed. But if you are not careful you can be "guilted" into doing *what other people think you should be doing.*

Family, friends, social commitments and holidays can be difficult for people who have fibromyalgia. Keep your priorities in check; volunteer your time and energy wisely during holidays and social events.

There is always a "Mrs. I-have-a-thousand-ways-you-should be-volunteering-your-time". You just have to graciously say "NO". Do not worry, she will find someone else to guilt into helping.

We do need organizers like that or things would probably not get done, but unfortunately, they are so good at their job and so used to listening to excuses from people that they tend to get rather pushy.

Do not worry about what people say about you "not doing enough for the family". Things like "doing Aunt Susie's housecleaning because she is 70 years old or visiting great aunt Sally who lives three hours away" should be handled in a way that you are physically capable of handling them.

It is important to take care of yourself and to spend the energy you have with your immediate family.

You could, for example, make a little extra for dinner occasionally or a little extra when baking cookies, and take or send the extra to aunt Susie; she will love it.

In addition, you could send an occasional "thinking of you" card to great aunt Sally and tuck in a picture of the children to let her know you are thinking about her at this holiday time.

Do not let people pressure you into doing things that are going to cause flare-ups or sap your strength. If that happened, who would take care of your family?

Make sure that aunt Susie understands why you cannot do her housekeeping and that it makes you feel badly for not being able to help.

Most of your friends and family will support you, but some may judge you in ignorance. Just assure them that you cannot always do everything you would like to do anymore, but that you will do what you can without jeopardizing your health.

After a while they will, hopefully, come to respect your limitations and support you.

Try to not let their attitudes stress you out. I know this is easier said than done, but if circumstances were reversed, you may not understand why a young, healthy-looking individual is not more active also.

Like us, our families are not perfect. So try to work with them to continue being a part of their lives. This can be very helpful for you in your efforts to maintain a healthy body and mind.

HOLIDAY COMMITMENTS

You can enjoy the holidays if you take care of yourself:

- When you are having family or friends over for dinner, do not be shy about asking for help or assigning tasks. Most people like to feel that they had a part in the festivities; they just need to be asked.

- If you are invited to a holiday get together, but you do not feel up to it, you can cordially decline by just explaining "you must pace yourself throughout the holidays as they are already starting to take a toll on you".

- If it is a holiday commitment that you just cannot get out of (especially if it's with extended family) perhaps the best way you can handle this is to prepare for it ahead of time.

  Plan on "taking it easy" for at least one or two days before and after the event. This does not necessarily mean "bed rest"; just relax your daily routine and take extra rest periods during your day.

- Be careful about taking on too many big projects, or making too many commitments and appointments at this time; remember your priorities.

- Prepare ahead for the possibility of the holidays taking a toll on your health by stocking up on a one week's supply of pre-frozen or "fast food" meals and using them as needed (Just try to pick the healthier pre-prepared foods).

- Pace yourself closely and do not spend more time on, or off, your feet than you should.

- Eat healthy in order to support your body's ability to keep up during this time of extra stress.

KEEPING THINGS SIMPLE

Keep things as uncomplicated as possible over the holidays, this includes holiday decorating. Below are some simple ideas that may get you started on your own plans for simplifying your holiday decorating and shopping woes.

- If you are going to have a large number of presents to wrap, some department stores still offer giftwrapping services.

  Check with local churches, schools and civic organizations; they may have gift wrapping services as fundraisers. If you or your neighbors have teenagers; they may gladly help wrap presents for some extra spending cash.

  Do not forget those wonderfully decorated bags and boxes

that you can just drop the gifts into with some brightly colored tissue paper and "voila" you are done.

- Shopping online is a great help during this time of year; you have a wider range of options, you can avoid a lot of the holiday hassle and can often save a little as well. The big advantage here is that it goes a long way in helping you avoid both mental and physical stress during this time of year.

- Decorating; let the kids do it and keep it simple. Remember, you may have to put it all away yourself and returning things to storage is usually much more time-consuming and exhausting than getting them out.

For some reason the holiday helpers who eagerly help to get things out to decorate are inevitably too busy with school etc. when it is time to put things away.

It may help to set a date that everything has to be back into storage because "When it's all done, we're going to see a movie" or "We're going to have a pizza and ice cream party" etc. You know what your family enjoys doing; use this as an incentive for helping you to get things put away before the holiday season is completely over and everyone gets settled into "life after the holidays".

- Here again, you may find others who are facing the same "after holiday cleanup blues" that would love to share this occasion by helping you and then having you help them rather than face the drudgery of doing it all alone.

- Mark everything well so next year there will be less hassle. Leave notes to yourself in the tops of the storage containers so you will not have unnecessary repeats of this year's problems.

REMEMBER THAT YOUR ENERGIES NEED TO BE SPENT ON THE THINGS THAT TOP YOUR PRIORITY LIST:

- Do not spend your holidays trying to impress everyone. This is an attitude that we should avoid year-round.

  How many times have you caused yourself to have miserable flare-ups just because you were trying to impress friends, associates or family?

- Live your life for those who are really important to you. Mary "so and so" of the "such and such" committee will not care about you three years down the road.

  Your husband, children, friends and grandchildren, will care about you even after you are gone from this life.

  So don't stress over "how to impress other people". Spend your energies being a part of your family's lives and their memories.

EMOTIONAL ROLLER COASTER

With fibromyalgia, as with any life-changing illness, you often find yourself on a roller coaster of emotional ups and downs.

You find yourself all set to do something you always enjoyed doing but your body does not want to cooperate.

You want to go places with your family, but you never know when fibromyalgia is going to spoil everybody's plans.

It can be very frustrating for you and for your family. if you are not careful this frustration could possibly lead to depression. This is one reason why it is important to take care of your health during holiday seasons.

VISITORS WITH CHILDREN

When visitors drop in over the holidays and bring their children with them, this can seem stressful for anyone who is not used to having children around; the best way to deal with this situation is to be prepared.

You may ask the parents to bring some of the child's favorite toys if you have nothing for them to play with. You may also ask them to bring some of their favorite snacks along.

If you wish to prepare for children visiting over the holidays, some simple snacks and something like kid friendly crackers, some little cheese squares or strips and maybe some small jars of peanut butter and natural jellies (rather than sugary ones) are good to keep on hand.

For sweet snacks, stay away from candy and sweet cookies with icing which tend to make children hyper. Instead, go for things like plain oatmeal cookies or graham crackers and milk. The parents will make up for anything else.

Have you ever had a neighbor to drop in over the holidays and bring their unruly child along? You watch in horror as the child runs around your house nonstop like a Tasmanian devil, ripping things out of drawers, knocking down precious items, yanking down decorations, trying to climb your curtains and terrorizing your pets?

All this time the parent acts as if the child is not even there. I have had this happen, and the best defense for this is a box of toys sitting discreetly behind a chair in the corner.

Many grandparents pick up used toys at yard sales, Goodwill or any other type of used goods stores. They take them home, clean them up and sanitize them for when the grandchildren come. Kids love to go through new toys or ones they have not seen for a while.

"My mother-in-law and father-in-law always kept a box of toys behind the recliner in the living room. I would also donate toys to the box that our children had outgrown or just seemed bored with."

They also had some board games that had been my husband's where they could be easily gotten to and a bucket of marbles and building blocks at the top of the stairs.

Within 15 minutes after entering their grandparents house all three children would be heard digging through "the box" and happily playing.

They also kept drawing tablets for the kids to draw on and plenty of crayons, pencils and coloring books.

While the grown-ups sat and talked, the kids would be at the table creating all sorts of works of art. When we were ready to leave, we and the kids all scouted the house for any toys that might have been left out of the box and made sure all art and craft items were put away.

There was no problem with kids roaming the house looking for things to get into. We always had a pleasant visit, and my kids will always have fond memories of going to grandma and grandpa's house.

Be honest with your family. If they support you and keep you as a part of their lives, there is a not a greater gift they could give you than to include you in their lives.

Let us all meet each

Other with a smile,

For the smile is the

Beginning of love.

Mother Teresa

****

The best thing to

Hold onto in life

Is each other.

Audrey Hepburn

****

CHAPTER 20
NATURAL SUPPLEMENTS AND HEALTHY CHANGES

Supplements are to be used to supplement a healthy diet; not to replace it.

Just as with prescribed medications, supplements alone are not the answer. It's equally important to pay attention to the diet and lifestyle changes that we discussed in this book. There is no one answer to reducing your symptoms; it just all works together, and you have to find out exactly what works best for you.

Before you take any form of pain relief or any other supplements suggested in this chapter, you should talk with your doctor and/or nutritionist. As I have stated before, every person is different and what helps one person may not be what is needed by another. You must also check the possibilities of interaction with any other health issues that you may have, prescribed medications you are taking and/or other supplements that you may be presently taking.

I have personally found that many of the same natural alternatives that are recommended for rheumatoid arthritis also are helpful for fibromyalgia pain. For those of us who suffer from both of these autoimmune disorders, this can definitely be a plus.

I am not a nutritionist, but through research, talking with various nutritionists, and trial and error, I have found these supplements to work quite well for me. I am sure that there are many other supplements that are helpful for pain and the many other symptoms of fibromyalgia. You should seek advice from a naturopathic doctor or a nutritionist before making any decision to use supplements to treat a medical problem.

SUPPLEMENTS FOR PAIN

Below, you will find a listing of supplements recommended in an article by the <u>Arthritis Foundation for RA</u>. I have found them to be very helpful for fibromyalgia pain as well.

1. **GINGER:** "Ginger has been shown to have anti-inflammatory properties similar to ibuprofen and CO X – 2 inhibitors. In a 2012 study, a specialized ginger extract reduced inflammatory reactions in rheumatoid arthritis as effectively as steroids did. Earlier studies show that taking a certain extract four times daily reduced osteoarthritis pain in the knee after three months of treatment, and another taken twice daily worked about as well as ibuprofen taken three times daily for hip and knee osteoarthritis pain."

2. **BOSWELLIA SERRATE:** "Has anti-inflammatory and analgesic (pain relieving) properties. It may also help inhibit the autoimmune process."

3. **CAPSAICIN** (from Chili peppers): "Temporarily reduces substance P, a pain transmitter. Its pain relieving properties have been shown in many studies, including a 2010 study published in Phytotherapy Research."

4. **TURMERIC/CURCUMIN**: "Curcumin is the chemical in turmeric that can reduce joint pain and swelling by blocking inflammatory cytokines and enzymes. A 2010 clinical trial using a turmeric supplement showed long-term improvement in pain and function in patients with knee osteoarthritis. A small 2012 study using a curcumin product showed more reduced joint pain and swelling in patients with active rheumatoid arthritis when compared to diclofenac sodium."

5. Avocado – Soybean Unsaponifiables (ASU):

"ASU blocks pro-inflammatory chemicals, prevents deterioration of synovial cells, which line joints, and may help regenerate normal connective tissue. A large three-year study published in 2013 showed that ASU significantly reduced progression of hip osteoarthritis. A 2008 meta-analysis found that ASU improved symptoms of hip and knee osteoarthritis and reduced or eliminated NSAID use." (I have not used this as of yet)

6. **Cat' s Claw** (the cat's claw must be free of tetra-cyclic oxindole alkaloids):

"Cat's Claw is an anti-inflammatory that inhibits tumor necrosis factor (TNF), a target of powerful rheumatoid arthritis drugs. It also contains compounds that may benefit the immune system. A small 2002 trial showed it reduced joint pain and swelling by more than 50 percent." (I have not tried this)

7. **Fish Oil: "Omega-3s** block anti-inflammatory cytokines and prostaglandins, and are converted by the body into powerful anti-inflammatory chemicals called resolvins. EPA and DHA have been extensively studied for rheumatoid arthritis and many other inflammatory conditions."

8. **Gamma Linolenic Acid** (use only cold-pressed, hexane free GLA):

"GLA is an Omega-6 fatty acid that the body converts into anti-inflammatory chemicals. In one trial, 56 patients with active rheumatoid arthritis showed significant improvement in joint pain, stiffness and grip strength after six months and progressive improvement in control of disease activity at one year. A smaller study found that a combination of GLA and fish oil significantly reduced the need for conventional pain relievers."

SUPPLEMENTS THAT I USE

Every person is different and that being said, please understand that I cannot recommend what is best for you. You should see a Naturopathic Doctor for a personal recommendation.

For muscle pain, I take magnesium (*best taken alone*), malic acid, plus the amino acids arginine or citrulline (*a supporter of arginine*) and lysine. But arginine and/or citrulline should not be taken within six hours of taking lysine because they use the same receptors and would cancel the lysine out.

I take a food-source multi-vitamin, a multi-mineral, and various anti-oxidants such as vitamin E, vitamin C, Alpha lipoic acid, CoQ10, resveratrol and astaxanthin. But supplements cannot replace the nutrients and benefits that you can get from a healthy diet. Supplements should only be used to supplement a healthy diet; not to replace it.

I eat a gluten-free, vegetarian diet rich in antioxidant fresh vegetables, fruits, herbs and spices. I also include Greek yogurt, Kefir, probiotics and prebiotics in my diet.

BRONCHITIS AND ASTHMA

These two problems often trouble many of us who have fibromyalgia.

For me, bronchitis was a seasonal problem; almost like clockwork, I would have a case of bronchitis every spring, fall and winter. I also had asthma from year-round allergies.

I was getting severe bronchitis on an average of four times a year.

Then one fall I just could not seem to shake the recurrence of bronchitis. My doctor prescribed an antibiotic and the bronchitis went away; 10 days after I had stopped taking the medication I had bronchitis again. Being as it was a weekend, I had to go to the emergency room and the doctor said the medication that he prescribed was the same medication he would prescribe for pneumonia.

Again, 10 days after I stopped taking the medication I had severe bronchitis again. My doctor had just left for an extended vacation so I went to a clinic. The doctor on duty prescribed an antibiotic and the bronchitis went away.

10 days after I stopped taking the medication I had bronchitis again. I returned to the clinic and the doctor told me that I could not keep taking these strong antibiotics. He said if I got bronchitis again he would not prescribe antibiotics for me; I would have to be admitted to the hospital.

Sure enough, 10 days after I stopped taking these antibiotics, I developed a severe case of bronchitis again. I was at my wits end; what was I going to do? I began researching everything I could find about bronchitis and natural alternatives. I finally happened upon a site that recommended Pau D' Arco for bronchitis.

At that time, there was very little information about Pau D' Arco. I had taken Pau D' Arco, in the past, for yeast infections because of its antifungal properties. I never thought of it being a natural antibiotic and an anti-inflammatory.

I opened two capsules, dumped the powder into a coffee cup, added hot water and honey and sipped on it; within an hour, my lungs were feeling better. I did this three to four times daily and a little over a week later, the bronchitis was gone and did not return.

From this time on, at the first hint of bronchitis, asthma or any difficulty taking a deep breath, I take Pau D' Arco. In the past ten years, I have only had one respiratory infection so severe that I had to be on antibiotics. This was following a time of extensive air-travel (need I say more?)

Pau D' Arco comes in capsules, teabags and tinctures. Drinking it as a tea or using the tincture is very soothing if I have a sore throat as well.

STRESS

Stress-related symptoms can often be helped by diet and supplements. One of the most helpful vitamins for stress is vitamin B. If you find vitamin B to cause digestive problems, there are alternatives to taking regular vitamin B supplements.

I have personally had a very serious problem with vitamin B in any form. I would take one dose and feel like I had the flu for 24 to 48 hours afterwards.

I have tried "B-50's, B-Complexes and multi-vitamins with vitamin B added"; I have used B tablets, capsules, liquids and gel-caps.

Through the years, I have tried "easily-digestible, time-released, and highly-absorbable vitamin B". I have taken them "before meals, in the middle of meals and after meals". I have taken them "with breakfast, with lunch and before dinner"; they all made me very ill.

My daughter suggested I try a vitamin B supplement recommended by her naturopathic doctor.

"B Stress", by Food Research, is a natural food supplement, not a mixture of synthetic vitamins like most vitamin B supplements are today. It did not make me ill and I felt a difference immediately.

For the first time in years, my body was actually receiving the benefits of this absolutely essential vitamin with no ill effects. I increase the dosage when I am under a lot of stress and find it makes it much easier to deal with stressful occurrences.

You can talk these suggestions over with your naturopathic doctor or nutritionist and hopefully work out a treatment plan for yourself.

Remember to include pacing, lifestyle changes, exercise programs, a healthy diet and therapies that have proven to help you as you set up your treatment plan.

I wish you well in your endeavors to lead a more productive and happy lifestyle. Be patient with your body and set realistic goals; given time, you will achieve them.

ABOUT THE AUTHOR

Alice Mowery Burnworth is a Kitchen and Bath Design Specialist and Co-author of "Stop the Yeast Syndrome Cookbook" with Dr. Morton Walker.

She currently resides in her country home in the North Eastern USA. As an internet researcher, researching documented information concerning autoimmune disorders, Alice has a website where she blogs information about concerns affecting fibromyalgia sufferers.

Alice's problems with autoimmune disorder began as a teenager, after contracting the Epstein-Barr virus. Immediately thereafter, she began to exhibit symptoms of Hypoglycemia, fatigue, Anemia and an abnormal sleep disorder similar to Narcolepsy. These symptoms have sporadically followed her throughout her adult life along with chronic Epstein-Barr flare-ups.

She also suffers from the symptoms of Rheumatoid Arthritis, Bursitis, Tendinitis, Fibromyalgia, Ehlers-Danlos, Hashimoto's Thyroiditis, IBS, Gluten Intolerance and Raynaud's Phenomenon. You are welcome to visit her fibromyalgia blog at: http://www.fibrozone.com/